Tuberculosis Control and Institutional Change in
Shanghai, 1911–2011

Tuberculosis Control and Institutional Change in Shanghai, 1911–2011

Rachel S. Core

Hong Kong University Press
The University of Hong Kong
Pok Fu Lam Road
Hong Kong
https://hkupress.hku.hk

© 2023 Hong Kong University Press

ISBN 978-988-8754-26-7 (*Hardback*)

All rights reserved. No portion of this publication may be reproduced or transmitted in any form or by any means, electronic or mechanical, including photocopying, recording, or any information storage or retrieval system, without prior permission in writing from the publisher.

British Library Cataloguing-in-Publication Data
A catalogue record for this book is available from the British Library.

Digitally printed

In memory of my teachers who inspired me to study China
Elisabeth Croll (1944–2007)
Roy Grow (1941–2013)
and Qiguang Zhao (1948–2015)

Contents

List of Illustrations	viii
List of Tables	ix
Acknowledgments	x
List of Acronyms	xiv
Note on Romanization	xvi
Introduction	1

Part I: Republican Era, 1911–1949

1. Tuberculosis and the Quest for Modernity in Shanghai, 1911–1927	25
2. An Unrealized Vision of Health and Tuberculosis Control, 1928–1949	46

Part II: Work-Unit Era, 1950–1992

3. Embracing a New Scientific Health Image in the Work Unit, 1950–1957	77
4. Shanghai's Great Leap Forward in Tuberculosis Control, 1958–1992	105
5. Building and Maintaining the Tuberculosis Control Network in Shanghai's Rural Counties, 1950s–1990s	127

Part III: Post-Work-Unit Era, 1992–2011

6. Dismantling of the Work-Unit System and Challenges to Tuberculosis Control in Shanghai, 1992–2011	151
Conclusion	177
Appendix: Tuberculosis Patient Interviewees	183
References	188
Index	208

Illustrations

Figure 0.1: Sanitation crew	2
Figure 0.2: Shanghai's population growth	15
Figure 0.3: Map of Shanghai	19
Figure 2.1: SATA's Shanghai Hospital	66
Figure 3.1: Shanghai's tuberculosis mortality rates	83
Figure 3.2: Respiratory disease transmission means	87
Figure 3.3: Anti-spitting poster	91
Figure 3.4: Anti-spitting poster	92
Figure 3.5: Mobile X-ray unit	97
Figure 3.6: Health and production are inseparable	98
Figure 4.1: Tuberculosis incidence for Yangpu District	110
Figure 6.1: Number of health-care institutions in Shanghai, 1978–2016	157

Tables

Table 0.1: Stages in tuberculosis development	9
Table 0.2: Characteristics of dominant systems in Shanghai	15
Table 1.1: Annual incidence of plague	36
Table 2.1: Deaths from communicable diseases in Shanghai's foreign concessions, 1937–1941	55
Table 3.1: Number of persons reached in TB educational programs	88
Table 3.2: Number of chest X-rays by institution	94
Table 5.1: Grassroots brigade implementation of the Cooperative Medical System, 1976	131
Table 6.1: Tuberculosis patient interviewees' characteristics	164

Acknowledgments

It is my honor and pleasure to thank the many individuals and institutions who supported this project, which was inspired by a discovery at the US National Library of Medicine (NLM). The NLM acquired the Chinese Public Health Collection (CPHC) around the time that I left China to begin graduate school in the United States. During the summer of 2007, I cataloged part of the CPHC, including a series of posters on tuberculosis. The series emphasized the importance of the state and workplace in making medical advances available—an opposite process from the one I witnessed when I was based in Chinese work units in 1998–2002. At the turn of the twenty-first century, Chinese citizens worried about mass layoffs, erosion of benefits, the growing cost of health care, and infectious disease control. China was in the throes of fundamental institutional change, which had profound implications for equity and global health.

This book began as a dissertation at The Johns Hopkins University. I am grateful for the guidance of my committee members and other sociology and East Asian studies faculty members. My dissertation supervisor, Joel Andreas, provided years of patient guidance and built a community of sociologists focusing on China. Marta Hanson introduced me to both the NLM's CPHC and a wider network of scholars working in the history of medicine in East Asia. Lingxin Hao joined my committee with the gusto and enthusiasm for research she brings to every conversation. Katherine Clegg Smith has been a proponent of qualitative methods in the health sciences and has continued to provide sage advice. Finally, Emily Agree joined the JHU Sociology Department at the most opportune time for a graduate student finishing a health-related dissertation. Other faculty who read drafts and offered advice include the late Mel Kohn, the late Giovanni Arrighi, Beverly Silver, Tobie Meyer-Fong, Kellee Tsai, Bill Rowe, Ho-Fung Hung, Huei-Ying Kuo, Stefanie DeLuca, Andy Cherlin, Karl Alexander, and Daniel Todes. My dissertation work was made possible by a number of grants, including summer travel grants from JHU's Institute for Global Studies and the Program in Cross-National Sociology and International Development in 2008 and from the East Asian Studies Program in 2009 and 2011. At JHU,

Acknowledgments xi

the following sociology and East Asian studies graduate students offered helpful feedback on various chapters and presentations of this work in progress: Dan Pasciuti, Shaohua Zhan, Ben Scully, Ke Ren, Ying Zhang, Lingli Huang, Yao Li, Yige Dong, Burak Gurel, Emily Mokros, and Jack Bandy.

Dissertation fieldwork during the 2010–2011 academic year was supported by a Fulbright Fellowship. I am grateful to the Chinese medical providers and healthcare recipients who shared their experience with me; these individuals must remain anonymous to protect their privacy. During my fieldwork and beyond, scholars at Fudan University, East China Normal University, and other institutions provided stimulating conversation, advice, and comradery. Those individuals include Tianshu Pan, Gao Xi, Zhang Letian, Cheng Yuan, Zhu Jianfeng, Guo Li, Shen Yifei, Dong Guoqiang, Wang Yan (Elly Wang), Jiang Jin, Zelin Yao, and Yulian Wu. During the time of my intensive document collection, Zhang Niumei provided research assistance. I am also grateful to my classmates and friends in the Hopkins-Nanjing Center alumni network who eased many trans-Pacific landings and helped me take (some) evenings off, including Chen Chen, Hsu Kun, Jia Min, Li Tong (Tommy), Lin Tao, Liu Zhan (Jerry), Luo Ying (Isa), Wang Qing, Wen Zhou, Weng Minjiang (Michael), Wu Jun (Julius), Xu Xi, Xu Yimei, and Zhao Hai. Desmond Fang, Emily Alitto Galbraith, David Erickson and Robert Price Jr. also deserve special mention for the friendship and laughter they provided.

My intellectual family has grown to a size where I cannot thank everyone individually. I am grateful to friends and colleagues working on sociology in China and in the history of medicine in East Asia who have offered helpful advice, including Bridie Andrews, Nicole Barnes, Mary Augusta Brazelton, Mary Bullock, Liping Bu, John DiMoia, James Flowers, Miriam Gross, Emily Hannum, Bian He, Lijing Jiang, Bill Johnston, Dorothy Ko, David Luesink, Cheiko Nakajima, Hilary Smith, Wayne Soon, Harry Wu, and Xun Zhou. I am also grateful for the comments that several friends have made to the proposal and chapter drafts: Felix Boeking, Xiaoping Fang, Tina Phillips Johnson, Yao Li, Nicole Mottier, Ruth Rogaski, Leander Seah, and Shi Xia.

At Stetson University, the Office of Academic Affairs, the College of Arts and Sciences Dean's Office, and the Brown Center for Faculty Innovation and Excellence have supported this project in many ways. I am grateful to Provosts Beth Paul and Noel Painter and Academic Affairs for supporting 2015, 2016, 2018, 2019, and 2022 summer grants, as well as a 2020–2021 sabbatical. The College of Arts and Sciences Dean's Office generously supported opportunities to present parts of this work at conferences in 2015–2022. The Brown Center sponsored Faculty Spotlights allowing me to present my research in January 2016, October 2019, and October 2021, as did the Asian studies program in November 2021. Colleagues, including Tony Abbott, Diane Everett, Tom Ferrell, Mayhill

Fowler, Eric Kurlander, Bill Nylen, Elizabeth Plantan, Rosalie Richards, Josh Rust, and Tara Schuwerk, have also supported the project in various ways. Sven Smith assumed summer chair duties, and Catherine Wright, Lauren Radesi, and Zaikeria Patha provided clerical support during final manuscript preparation.

When I was (remote) scholar-in-residence through New York University's Faculty Resource Network (FRN) in the fall of 2020, the FRN staff, Rebecca Karl, Christiana Coyle, and Beth Katzoff provided advice and support. In the spring and summer of 2021, Taiwan's Ministry of Foreign Affairs supported my final seven months of sabbatical with a Taiwan Fellowship. I am grateful to the staff of the Center for Chinese Studies and the National Central Library for their support, and to the Academia Sinica's Institute of Modern History (IMH) for serving as my host institution. From before I was released from quarantine, Sean Hsiang-lin Lei, Mike Shiyung Liu, and Shu-ching Chang made me feel welcome. Well-attended talks, in person at the IMH and virtually for Taiwan Fellowship recipients, helped me to clarify parts of the manuscript. I am grateful for suggestions and advice from many scholars, including Chen Yung-fa, Evan Dawley, Paul Katz, Wen-Hua Kuo, Shang-jen Li, Shao-hao Liu, Arukwe Nnannan Onuoha, Mårten Söderblom Saarela, Wen-ti Comet Song, Chuck Wooldridge, Sandy Xu, and Ning Jennifer Zhang.

Librarians at JHU's Milton S. Eisenhower Library, the Shanghai Library, and the Shanghai Municipal Archives have helped me track down many useful materials. At JHU, Ellen Keith, Yuanyuan Zeng, and Yunshan Ye were especially helpful. Stetson's duPont-Ball Library staff have handled my many requests over the past eight years. Special mention goes to Barbara Costello and the Inter-Library Loan staff who have helped to get titles with alacrity. In Taiwan, staff at the IMH's Kuo Ting-yee Library approached my requests with patience and good cheer. Final research for this book was conducted at the Library of Congress and was facilitated by the staff of the Asian Reading Room, and especially Yuwu Song.

I am grateful to the staff at Hong Kong University Press for shepherding this project, as well as for the helpful suggestions by two anonymous reviewers. All mistakes and omissions in this book are entirely my own.

Parts of this book draw upon previously published work. I am grateful to the Indiana University Press, Springer Nature, and the *American Journal of Chinese Studies* for allowing me to adapt copyrighted materials. Parts of Chapters 2, 3, 4, and 6 revisit arguments made in three previously published works: "Tuberculosis Control in Shanghai: Bringing Health to the Masses, 1928–Present," published in the 2014 volume *Medical Transitions in Twentieth-Century China*, edited by Bridie Andrews and Mary Brown Bullock (Bloomington: Indiana University Press); "The Fall and Rise of Tuberculosis: How Institutional Change Affected Health Outcomes in Shanghai, 1927–2013," in the *Fudan Journal of Humanities and Social Sciences* 9: 65–90, 2015; and "Institutional Change and Tuberculosis

Control: Continuity and Change in Pre- and Post-1949 Shanghai" in *AJCS* 26(2): 73–89, October 2019.

On a personal note, I am grateful for the balance that gyms and trainers in Baltimore, Shanghai, Singapore, and DeLand, have provided. Special mention goes to Jen Horton, Marta Ash Enders, and Laura Collette for providing high-intensity classes to counter the toughest writing days. In Taiwan, during the 73-day level-3 COVID-19 shutdown, Will Sima, and Ivy Kwek helped this gym rat discover that mountains and bike paths are far more scenic than the group exercise studio, a habit I have avidly continued in Florida (without the mountains). Finally, I am grateful to Brian McNamara for putting up with my megalomaniacal quest to finish this book and for making me laugh every day. This book is dedicated to the two late Carleton College professors who led my first study abroad adventures in China, Qiguang Zhao and Roy Grow, and to my late mentor at SOAS, Lisa Croll.

Acronyms

ACF	active case finding
AIDS	acquired immunodeficiency syndrome
BCG	bacillus Calmette-Guérin (anti-tuberculosis vaccine)
BFD	barefoot doctor
BHO	branch health office
CCP	Chinese Communist Party
CDC	Center for Disease Control
CHC	Community Health Center
CMA	China Medical Association
CMB	China Medical Board
CMMA	China Medical Missionary Association
CMS	Cooperative Medical System
COE	collectively owned enterprises
CPHC	Chinese Public Health Collection
DOTS	Direct Observed Therapy, short-course
FMC	French Municipal Council
GDP	gross domestic product
GIS	government insurance system
GLF	Great Leap Forward
GMD	Guomindang
GVIO	gross value of industrial output
HDI	human-development index
HIV	human immunodeficiency virus
HOR	*Health Officer's Report*

INH	isoniazid
IPT	isoniazid preventive therapy
LIS	labor insurance system
MDR	multidrug resistant
NATAC	National Anti-Tuberculosis Association of China
NLM	National Library of Medicine
NTA	National Tuberculosis Association (US)
PH	public health
PRC	People's Republic of China
PUMC	Peking Union Medical College
R	rifampin
RMB	renminbi, a unit of currency equivalent to one yuan
S	streptomycin
SARS	severe acute respiratory syndrome
SATA	Shanghai Anti-Tuberculosis Association
SEZ	special economic zone
SMA	Shanghai Municipal Archives
SMC	Shanghai Municipal Council
SOE	state-owned enterprise
TB	tuberculosis
TVE	township and village enterprise
UK	United Kingdom
US	United States
USD	United States dollar
WHO	World Health Organization
WTO	World Trade Organization
WUS	work-unit system
XDR	extremely drug resistant
YMCA	Young Men's Christian Association

Note on Romanization

This work spans a full century, during which more than one transliteration system was used for Chinese. Because the bulk of the chapters cover post-1949, I make use of the *hanyu pinyin* system to romanize most words and phrases. The exception to this rule is names of prominent figures—for example, Sun Yat-sen—for whom the Wade-Giles or alternative transliteration is most widely known. Because the text focuses on mainland China, simplified Chinese characters are used in places to clarify the original text/meaning. All translations are my own.

Introduction

A public health (PH) poster from China depicts some of the steps for sanitizing the room where an infectious respiratory disease sufferer has stayed before another patient can occupy the same space. The image shows three members of a housekeeping crew. The crew members are not in hazmat suits, but they do wear personal protective equipment: full-length white coats, hair coverings, and white face masks. The windows are open to let in fresh air and sunlight in an attempt to kill or disperse microorganisms. The worker closest to the window stands in a sunbeam as they wipe down the surface of a table. In the foreground, one worker mops the floor while another sprays disinfectant from a tank on their back. While these sanitation workers may make contemporary viewers think of efforts to control COVID-19, or the severe acute respiratory syndrome (SARS) in 2002–2003, they actually attempted to control another airborne microorganism: the tuberculosis (TB) bacillus. The poster is one of a series of 30 public health posters created for a 1953–1954 exhibit by the Shanghai Anti-Tuberculosis Association (SATA, 上海防痨协会).

Like recent global pandemics, pulmonary tuberculosis is a respiratory disease, transmitted through microscopic droplets. These droplets are released into the atmosphere when a person with active disease coughs, and infection occurs by inhaling the droplets. Like COVID-19, tuberculosis outbreaks expose social inequities and trends. For instance, like COVID-19, TB disproportionately affects the poor, who often live in crowded conditions and may face malnutrition. Poor people, including migrants, might be unable to take time off work, either because their jobs are deemed "essential" to the food, health, or transportation system, or because they simply cannot afford to miss a paycheck. Like COVID-19, TB disproportionately affects vulnerable populations—prisoners, persons with preexisting conditions (such as diabetes), immunocompromised individuals, and the elderly. Like COVID-19, TB can be stigmatizing, making affected individuals or the geographical region where they reside the source of ridicule or blame. Likewise, some of the same public health protocols enacted to control TB's spread—for example, widespread case identification and physical isolation—can also be used to control COVID-19.

Figure 0.1: Sanitation crew

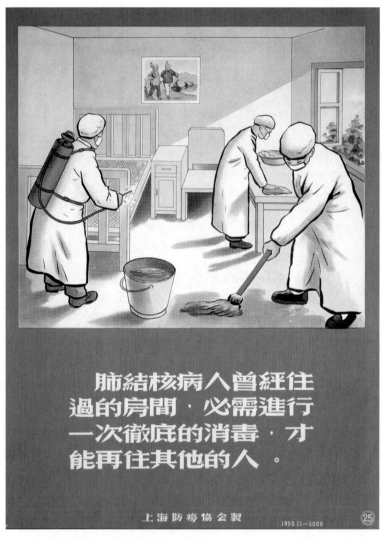

SATA 1953. The poster reads: "The room where a person infected with TB stayed should be thoroughly sterilized before anyone else is permitted to stay there." Courtesy of the United States National Library of Medicine.

Introduction

Unlike emerging infectious diseases, humanity has been concerned with tuberculosis for centuries. In 1882, Robert Koch's discovery of the TB bacillus catalyzed a decades-long struggle to interrupt transmission until effective antibiotics were discovered in the 1940s and 1950s. Interruption of transmission took place largely by isolating persons with active disease, either in sanatoria or at home. By the 1950s, discovery of antibiotics quelled the need for isolation; however, as the rollout of the COVID-19 vaccine in many parts of the world has illustrated, an effective distribution system is key to a society's ability to take advantage of biomedical advances. Despite the existence of effective antibiotics for 70 years, TB remained the world's leading cause of death from respiratory disease through 2019, with more than 1 million people dying each year (WHO 2019).[1] Alarmingly, the past four decades have seen tuberculosis resurgence, including in global cities, where shiny exteriors mask the unequal conditions many essential workers face.

TB has also been the leading infectious disease in China, both historically and today. This book investigates how tuberculosis was managed effectively starting in the 1950s and why it became a major health concern, again, precisely during the time that China's economic might was growing, in the 1990s and early 2000s. The decline of TB in China coincided with the creation and maintenance of the work-unit (单位) system (WUS), and the recent TB control challenges have coincided with the dismantling of this system. This is more than a coincidence. This book demonstrates the critical role the work-unit system played in making medical advances available and that its dismantling was an important factor in TB control challenges between 1992 and 2010. Under the work-unit system, created during the 1950s, the vast majority of urban residents had guaranteed employment, with a host of benefits tied to their workplace, and there was little mobility. This system gave urban residents access to food, housing, and health care through their workplace. While the term "work-unit system" is often used to denote only the urban system, in this book, I also investigate rural production brigades created under collectivization in Shanghai's surrounding counties because they performed similar functions. Work units played a key role in China's TB control because they were the delivery point for medical and public health services. In the 1980s, the rural cooperative medical system was dismantled in much of China. The urban work-unit-based health-access system was dismantled in the 1990s. In the 1980s and 1990s, the rise of temporary and casual employment gave rise to a huge population of migrant workers, who had few rights in their receiving areas, including limited access to health care. The decline of the work-unit system was a critical factor that has led to the TB control challenges China faced in recent decades.

---

1. Since 2020, COVID-19 has outstripped TB as the deadliest infectious disease worldwide.

Institutional Change, Public Health, and Modernization in China

A host of recent scholarship has demonstrated that health was a central concern of each successive Chinese government as part of twentieth-century modernization (Yip 1995; Rogaski 2004; Andrews 2014; Lei 2014; Bu 2017; Baum 2018; N. E. Barnes 2018; Brazelton 2019b). In the past century, each Chinese government has adopted some of the health and infection control protocols enacted by the previous government(s), as well as some of its own. Many of these health and infection protocols have also been informed by China's international alliances, which differed dramatically depending on the party in power. This book is organized around three periods corresponding with different government orientations: before 1949, 1950–1992, and after 1992. The importance of 1949 as a temporal dividing line will be obvious to those familiar with Chinese history: in 1949, the Chinese Communist Party (CCP) founded the People's Republic of China (PRC). The choice of 1992 as a critical juncture may be less obvious. Some readers will, no doubt, wonder why 1992 was chosen, instead of 1978, when the era of economic reform began. Certainly, some institutional change occurred as initial market reforms were introduced starting in 1978, particularly in rural areas; however, prior to 1992, Chinese leaders hotly debated the direction of future reforms (Shirk 1993). Only with Deng Xiaoping's Southern Tour to the special economic zones (SEZs) of Shenzhen and Zhuhai, as well as Shanghai in 1992, was the future direction of China's economic development set: China would fully embrace more capitalist-style market reforms.

Prior to 1949, state and other actors made some attempts at health-care provision and TB control, and both 1911 and 1928 were key moments. The 1910–1911 Manchurian plague catalyzed the modern Chinese state to create some public health infrastructure and protocols, such as the isolation of respiratory disease sufferers. Starting in 1928, the Guomindang (GMD, 国民党) believed the state should provide health and welfare services, thereby strengthening citizenship and the nation (M. L. Bian 2005; Dillon 2015). After the GMD came to power, political power in China remained highly decentralized, and one way the GMD aimed to unify the nation was by promoting the National Health Reconstruction program, informed by nineteenth-century health movements in Europe and the United States, which were largely concerned with sanitation and identifying the organisms responsible for spreading disease (Rosen 1993).[2]

The GMD started to implement its vision during the 1928–1937 Nanjing Decade; however, from 1937 to 1945, the War of Resistance against the Japanese

---

2. Rosen notes a shift from the sanitation era—which was largely concerned with creating infrastructure for water and waste—to the bacteriological era in the late nineteenth century. Discovery of the microorganisms that caused diseases such as diphtheria and tuberculosis ushered in the second era and the predominance of the germ theory of disease.

Introduction 5

compromised the state's ability to deliver on parts of this vision, such as health promotion. While the post-1949 Communist government aimed to distance itself from the previous administration including with respect to its approach to health, recent scholarship has rooted the Communist ability to implement widescale health advances after 1949 to efforts during the war (Barnes and Watt 2014; N. E. Barnes 2018; Brazelton 2019b; Soon 2020). As Nicole Barnes (2022) has demonstrated, the dictum "Serve the People" (为人服务)—a hallmark of the Mao era—can be used to describe the actions of female doctors, nurses, and midwives between 1937 and 1945. Before 1949, the first steps were taken to create health institutions, such as TB hospitals, but many facilities were run by nonprofits, rather than the state. Indeed, institutional commitment to providing care to the wider population was slower to develop; change would come with other political and economic transformation.

After the CCP came to power in 1949, its socialist modernization program included several components: the state was to plan the economy, employ everybody, and take responsibility for everyone's welfare, including their health. Under this paradigm, every locale was reorganized according to the work-unit system, which tied individuals to production units, provided services via these units, and immobilized the population. In urban areas, most formal-sector places of employment—factories, schools, hospitals and other healthcare institutions, commercial and cultural enterprises, banks, transportation infrastructure such as train stations and bus depots, and so on—were reorganized as work units. By 1957, almost all urban Chinese adults were expected to be employed in one of these units, but this ideal was never fully achieved. Indeed, most urban youth subsequently entered the work-unit system through a standard path: upon graduation from middle school or college, they were assigned to a unit. Ideally, they remained for the duration of their working years, until they retired. In reality, full employment in urban areas was never universal, but provision of social welfare benefits was premised on inclusion in the system.

Creation of the work-unit system did two important things with respect to health. First, it established a system of workplace-based entitlements that became known as the "iron rice bowl." Chinese workers depended more on work units socially and economically than most Westerners ever depended on their workplaces. Work units approved or disapproved marriages and provided civil, educational, and health services formerly carried out by the family. In addition to salaries, urban work units distributed food coupons, subsidized cafeterias and housing, and provided family planning, daycare, education and vocational training for workers, and schooling for workers' children. By providing food and housing, work units mitigated some of the underlying factors associated with the development of disease. Because employees of work units often lived and worked together, spending considerable time in these relatively isolated cellular units, work units might be considered "total institutions."[3] Most pertinent to this book, work units provided medical insurance and primary health care and served as the workers' principal access point to the medical and public health systems (Henderson and Cohen 1984). Larger work units even had attached hospitals or clinics.

In rural areas, a similar process of agricultural collectivization and provision of social services occurred, starting in the early 1950s. As in urban areas, rural production brigades eventually provided their members with medical insurance and primary health care and served as workers' principal access point to the medical and public health systems; however, the cooperative medical system (CMS) was not created until about a decade after the health system was established in urban areas. While some rural areas developed health infrastructure earlier, the CMS arose in response to the health crisis of the 1958–1961 Great Leap Forward (Zhou 2020). Starting in the 1960s, most brigades also had a health clinic staffed by one or more health paraprofessionals, who became known as "barefoot doctors." In the 1970s, a wave of scholarly publications examined China's rural health system; some even argued it could become a low-cost model for infectious disease control in other countries (Horn 1971; Pickowicz 1971; V. W. Sidel and R. Sidel 1974; V. H. Li 1975; New and New 1975; R. Sidel and V. W. Sidel 1977; Rifkin 1978). This system was a huge improvement because it brought some medical care and public health education to rural areas, but it had a host of problems, such as poorly trained health workers who were overreliant on Western medicine. There was also wide variation among what rural communes themselves could provide, the system was inferior to the urban system, and there were great disparities between what was provided between coastal and interior provinces.

From a disease control standpoint, a major change after 1949 was ensuring that medical and public health advances, such as case-finding efforts and effective antibiotics, reached the masses. Along with schistosomiasis, sexually transmitted infections, and cholera, TB was one of the targeted infectious diseases that helped to shape public health policy in the early Mao era (Gross 2016; Fang 2021). Despite China's exclusion from many organizations, including the World Health Organization, during the Mao era, the nation's control model emphasized the same prevention and case-finding methods used elsewhere in the world, along with an improved TB control network and more effective TB drugs. Work units facilitated public health education and TB case finding and paid the cost of TB treatment. Workplace doctors, in both urban and rural areas, supervised treatment, monitoring compliance with treatment regimens. Thus, because the

---

3. Sociologist Erving Goffman defined total institutions as places in which similarly situated individuals live, largely cut off from wider society (1961).

Introduction

work-unit system was intrusive, premised on social control, it could effectively squelch infectious disease outbreaks.

Starting in the 1980s, rural production brigades were dismantled, which affected the CMS, but rural industrial enterprises owned by villages and townships expanded rapidly and still provided support for some rural health-care provision, especially in the areas of coastal China, where they were most widespread. In cities, the work-unit and residence permit (户口) systems remained in place, with public ownership and permanent employment, as well as work-unit-based provision of welfare and health care. Because of this, there was little room for migrant labor until the 1990s.

After 1990, the CCP's new capitalist-style market reform program, based on market integration and profit-oriented enterprises, dismantled the work-unit system, cut the ties between the enterprise and individuals, spurred mobility, and dismantled the basic-level health-care and public health system that had been based in these units. This took place gradually, as the Chinese government restructured state-owned enterprises (SOEs) and collective enterprises. Most SOE and collective enterprises were privatized, and those remaining were reorganized.[4] In an attempt to increase the competitiveness of SOEs and collectives, restructuring required enterprises to shed their employment guarantees and welfare functions. Many work-unit clinics and hospitals were privatized or eliminated. As permanent employment ended, temporary and casual employment became common.

The decline of the work-unit system led to a crisis of public health, health insurance, and provision of care from the 1980s to 2010s. The amount of coverage provided through the workplace declined, and urban and rural residents were expected to pay for care at the time services were rendered (Wong, Lo, and Tang 2006). Municipal governments in China began to replace lost health insurance in the early 2000s, but coverage remained limited until around 2010. Starting in 2006, the state also began to rebuild a new cooperative medical system (NCMS), but coverage was not as complete as under the original CMS. In 2011, the Chinese minister of health, a former barefoot doctor, reported that out-of-pocket expenses for rural residents who had joined the NCMS had fallen from 73.4 percent to 49.5 percent in three years (Watts 2008; Z. Chen 2011), which still proved burdensome to many rural residents.

Work-unit dismantling in the 1990s also led to declining access to tuberculosis control interventions. On paper, access to tuberculosis treatment should have been widespread, given that the World Health Organization began to widely

---

4. A few types of work units, such as government agencies and enterprises in the energy sector, have retained important elements of the work-unit system, but these make up a relatively small portion of the labor force.

promote a free, six-month course of medication following the declaration of TB as a global health emergency in 1993. However, in China, health educational programs and case finding were done less frequently in workplaces than they were under the work-unit system. Patients no longer received TB treatment in a workplace-based clinic under the supervision of workplace doctors. This study demonstrates how these changes led to TB control challenges. The lessons from several decades of institutional change in China are also important to controlling other infectious diseases. In recent times, resurgence and emergence of new pathogens has demonstrated that continued vigilance toward infectious diseases is necessary. As the first pandemic of the new millennium, SARS attracted attention to China's health system, which had become fragmented in the 1980s and 1990s. Scholars have argued that SARS served as a wake-up call, which led to the reprioritization of public health in China in the contemporary era (S. Wang 2004; Mason 2016).

The Fall and Return of Tuberculosis in the Twentieth Century

Tuberculosis is one of the key diseases for illustrating the importance of social factors in disease control. Globally, both the decline of tuberculosis in the twentieth century and TB control challenges in recent decades came about because of a number of variables. The goal of TB control, both historically and in the present day, is to lower the number of cases and deaths by interrupting disease transmission and progression, which may take place at any stage of disease development, from infection to death (Table 0.1). Interventions designed to prevent the body from being infected by the TB bacillus include social distancing, education about transmission and symptoms, as well as the widespread use of the bacillus Calmette-Guérin (BCG) vaccine.[5] Interventions to prevent the body's breakdown into active disease aim to keep the immune system strong. Only a small percent of individuals infected by the TB bacillus ever develop active disease. Those who do often have compromised immune systems—either caused by malnutrition or the human immunodeficiency virus (HIV) / acquired immunodeficiency syndrome (AIDS). In contemporary times, isoniazid preventive therapy (IPT) can also be employed to prevent active disease from ever developing.[6] During

---

5. Prepared from a weakened strain of bovine TB, BCG came into extended use worldwide in the years following World War II. Compared to other childhood vaccines, such as the MMR vaccine against measles, mumps, and rubella, which offers more than 90 percent effectiveness, BCG's effectiveness is not as robust. It is most effective in providing resistance against disseminated TB—a condition where TB spreads throughout the body—among children, than against pulmonary TB in adults (Davenne and McShane 2016).

6. IPT entails taking one of the most effective TB drug for a course of six months, which prevents latent TB from ever becoming active.

Introduction

Table 0.1: Stages in tuberculosis development

	Infection risk	Breakdown risk	Death risk
Direct causes	Breathing in the TB bacillus	Immunosuppressive event	Lack of appropriate treatment
Proximate causes	Coughing without covering the mouth	Inadequate nutrition	Diagnosis delays
	Poorly ventilated environments	Nonadherence to IPT	Treatment nonadherence
	Lack of exposure to sunlight	Unsafe sexual behavior	
	Failure to get the BCG vaccine		
Underlying causes	Overcrowding	Lack of money for a nutritious diet	Lack of access to health care
		Lack of health education	
		Lack of AIDS knowledge	

Adapted from Jaramillo (1999).

the final stage of disease development, interventions are made to find and treat persons with active disease to prevent death, by identifying cases and managing active TB through rest and drug therapy.

The TB development stages outlined in Table 0.1 also distinguish among the direct, proximate, and underlying causes of disease. The direct causes are all biomedical factors; however, these factors cannot be separated from the proximate and underlying factors. The proximate causes of disease include many behavioral factors, such as failure to get or adhere to (preventive) treatment(s). Behavioral factors often interrelate with more distal-level factors, or underlying causes—what sociologists refer to as the social determinants, or fundamental causes, of disease (Link and Phelan 1995; Marmott 2004; Navarro 2007). In the United States and the UK, race is among the most important of the social determinants of health, but this monograph primarily investigates variables other than race.[7] Specifically, socioeconomic class and structural divisions associated with inclusion in and exclusion from the work-unit system are the primary variables of importance. Economic standing enables or limits individual compliance with public health and medical recommendations. For instance, poor people are more

---

7. As Chapters 1 and 2 will discuss, race was a factor that played into policies by colonial governments and nonprofits prior to 1942.

likely to live in crowded housing or food deserts, where they are unable to maintain a balanced diet. Likewise, poor areas may have more limited educational opportunities, including on the subject of health. Poor people might lack access to preventive technologies, such as BCG, IPT, or even condoms. Moreover, as a disease develops, poor people might delay care seeking, either because they lack insurance or because they are unable to take time off work. Equally important to the analysis in this book are structural divisions. In China, inclusion in an urban or rural workplace also influenced one's residence permit status (*hukou*) and accompanying benefits allocation.[8]

Many of the factors identified in Table 0.1 were important both to the historical spread of TB as well as to new challenges to TB control in recent decades. Historically, discovery of effective antibiotics was a game changer for TB control, causing it to decline rapidly in the 1950s–1970s. However, as noted above, after discovery of effective biomedical advances, they must be distributed among the population. Prior to the discovery of effective antibiotics—streptomycin (S) in 1943 and isoniazid (H/INH) in 1952—chemical means of interrupting disease progression had not been proven. Consequently, interventions often aimed to either raise standards of living or to prevent initial transmission. As a result, TB infection and death rates declined in many places throughout the globe, including Shanghai, even prior to the discovery of antibiotics.[9]

Scholars have been divided regarding which factors were key to this decline. While Thomas McKeown (1976) has emphasized how rising standards of living improved nutrition, the social interventions emphasized by his critics, such as isolating TB sufferers in sanatoria, were also critically important (Szreter 1988). Economic resources limit the range of public health interventions possible. At the macro level, economic resources include investment in the public health and health-care systems, potentially including commitment to universal healthcare. The micro level includes factors that are still relevant to COVID-19: inability to socially distance, whether at home or work, malnutrition, and diagnosis delays. In recent decades, the scattered voices emphasizing poverty as a leading cause of disease have started to form a chorus (D. S. Barnes 1995; Farmer 1997, 2001).

As multiple factors contributed to the decline of tuberculosis both before antibiotic discovery and after, multiple factors have been responsible for the

---

8. Alexander and Chan (2004) have likened the urban-rural exclusion established under the *hukou* to apartheid.

9. For falling TB in Beijing, Shanghai, and Guangdong, see Zhang and Elvin (1998). Likewise, Bill Johnston (1995) examines government interventions in Japan. Lynda Bryder (1988) investigates the social factors contributing to TB in England, Randall Packard (1989) in South Africa, and David Barnes (1995) in Paris. Barbara Bates (1992), Sheila Rothman (1994), Georgina Feldberg (1995), Katherine Ott (1996), Samuel Kelton Roberts Jr. (2009), and Christian McMillen (2015) have all examined the social determinants of health in America. Packard, Bates, Feldberg, Ott, Roberts, and McMillen particularly consider race as an important variable.

resurgence of TB in recent decades, for example, the emergence of HIV/AIDS and of multidrug-resistant (MDR) TB, migration, and the dismantling of health systems, often with more than one variable interacting. Some of the factors driving the global resurgence of TB are relevant to China, but others have more limited relevance. For instance, while HIV/AIDS is arguably the most important factor driving resurgent TB in Sub-Saharan Africa, prevalence in China is not as high. Since China began more widespread HIV/AIDS messaging in the early 2000s, it has been relatively successful in preventing HIV from becoming a generalized infection, with heterosexual contact as a primary transmission means (Anagnost 2007; Hyde 2007; S.-h. Liu 2011; WHO 2019). HIV/AIDS in China has disproportionately affected higher-risk groups, leading to their stigmatization: intravenous drug users in the border areas of Xinjiang and Yunnan, impoverished peasants who sold their plasma and were infected with contaminated blood in Henan, men who have sex with men, and sex workers. Nevertheless, increased incidence of syphilis in China's most developed regions suggests cause for concern regarding heterosexually transmitted infections (Chen et al. 2007; Tucker, Chen, and Peeling 2010; Henderson et al. 2014).

The emergence of a disproportionately high number of MDR cases is an important part of China's TB resurgence. MDR-TB is defined as TB that is resistant to at least two of the most commonly used drugs, isoniazid and rifampin (R).[10] According to the 2000 All-China Epidemiological Study of Tuberculosis Prevalence, an estimated 1 in 10 cases was infected with a drug-resistant strain. In the early 2000s, China had one-third of the world's burden of MDR-TB cases (Wang, Liu, and Chin 2007; Zhao et al. 2012; Long, Qu, and Lucas 2016). Countries in eastern Europe saw increased incidence of MDR-TB, driven by the collapse of their socialist systems (Borgdorff, Floyd, and Broekmans 2002; Koch 2013). The disproportionate load of MDR cases in China is more paradoxical because other health indicators, such as life expectancy, have continued to rise in China, while they have fallen in some eastern European countries (Cockerham 1999; McKee 2005; Stuckler, King, and McKee 2009).

Drug resistance may have originally arisen largely from noncompliance with drug therapy, but this question is complex. Drug resistance develops not just because of irresponsible, willful patients but also because of imperfect science and unequal access to treatment. Drug resistance has existed for almost as long as effective TB antibiotics. Shortly after streptomycin was discovered, research recognized the potential for the development of resistant strains. By the late 1940s, para-aminosalicylic acid was used in combination with streptomycin in an attempt to prevent the development of streptomycin-resistant disease strains.

---

10. Extremely drug resistant (XDR)-TB is TB that is resistant to H, R, a fluoroquinolone, and one of three injectable drugs: capreomycin, kanamycin, and amikacin (Ghandi et al. 2010).

Despite the fact that these natural mutations in the microorganism might cause multidrug-resistant strains, patients have taken much of the blame because noncompliance with treatment regimens can also lead to drug resistance.

The issue of compliance with medical recommendations has a complex history. Patients might be noncompliant for any number of reasons, including lack of understanding, lack of resources, or because the medicine they are taking makes them feel worse rather than better. In many cases, patients are not willfully noncompliant; their noncompliance results from an inability to obtain TB medicines due to problems in the supply chain, inadequate medical access, or poverty (Okeke, Lamikanra, and Edelman 1999). Paul Farmer's work on TB and HIV/AIDS coinfection in Haiti considers the question of noncompliance and its inevitability among the poor. Farmer argues that we must question whether the term "noncompliant" is even useful "in describing the experience of a young man whose family was willing to sell its land to treat him" (Farmer 1997: 351–52). Farmer uses the term "new TB" to highlight that the two ostensibly biological factors central to it—drug-resistant strains and the advent of HIV—are best understood as "sociomedical phenomena" brought on by social forces such as poverty and economic inequality.

Migration is also a factor driving faltering TB control in many countries worldwide, including China (Frieden et al. 1995; Festenstein and Grange 1999; Fujiwara 2000; M.-J. Ho 2004; Enarson 2006; Cain et al. 2008). Persons who migrate voluntarily are often pushed from declining opportunities in sending areas and pulled by increasing opportunities—or at least perceived opportunities—in receiving areas. In receiving areas, migrants often live and work in poor conditions, making them more susceptible to TB and other infectious diseases, and also frequently lack health insurance or regular access to the health system. The communication, quality-of-life, and health access challenges Chinese rural-to-urban migrants face are similar to those international migrants face globally (Wang et al. 2007; Wei et al. 2009; Chen et al. 2013). Other studies have found much higher success in managing TB treatment among urban permanent residents than among peasant migrants in China (Zhang et al. 2006; Shen et al. 2012; Xue et al. 2018). These trends suggest discrepancies in exposure as well as health access issues, both of which relate to the decline of the work-unit system, which served to limit exposure and increase access. Migrants often have the least access to clinics that provide primary care. Moreover, prior to 2004, they were not entitled to free TB treatment in their receiving areas (Lu et al. 2020).

Changes to health and public health delivery systems are also part of the explanation for TB challenges in China, and this factor will be central to the analysis in this book. Changes to health-care and public health delivery systems, increase TB by limiting access to health services. In many countries, these changes involve privatization, which has been part of a larger neoliberal (i.e., market-driven) agenda since the 1980s. In the health-care sector, the neoliberal approach has included implementation of a fee-for-service model at many places around the globe.[11] This factor has been especially important in postsocialist countries, many of which have seen increased TB incidence and mortality (Borgdorff, Floyd, and Broekmans 2002; Altman 2008; Beaubien 2013; Koch 2013). Stuckler, King, and McKee (2009) showed a link between the privatization of SOEs and increased mortality generally in postsocialist European countries (406). While scholars have not always articulated the causal mechanisms through which privatization and increased unemployment might lead to rising disease, Erin Koch's 2013 ethnography on post-Soviet Georgia helped to illustrate the interaction between disruption of social services, such as preventive health care, poverty, and the movement of people. Likewise, Keshavjee (2014) investigates retrenchment and neglect of health programs in former Soviet republics. Keshavjee engages most explicitly with the effect of neoliberalism on health, highlighting the implosion of life expectancy in Tajikistan.

Much attention has been paid to the collapse of the health system in China's countryside. This system was largely dismantled in the 1980s, and scholars have concerned themselves with how the transformation of China's rural health system has led patients to delay seeking health care, stop treatment, or forego care entirely because of the prohibitive cost (Henderson and Cohen 1984; Henderson et al. 1994; S. Wang 2004). Scholars have not paid as much attention to the health effects of work-unit system reforms in urban areas, even though social scientists have studied its other social effects.[12] Scholars who have investigated the effect of urban economic reforms on health care have often focused on changes in the insurance system, though scholars have grown increasingly attentive to the health effects of structural reforms in recent years (Duckett 2004; Wong, Lo, and Tang 2006).

Chinese economic and health reforms have occurred within a wider set of neoliberal reforms occurring globally, and many of China's efforts resemble those introduced elsewhere. Privatization is a large part of this model, and it includes both entities in the industrial and financial sectors, as well as the health sector. Privatization of some industries has led to widening inequalities, both within regions and between regions, and these inequalities also manifest in health inequalities, such as widening gaps in life expectancy between provinces. China

---

11. In 1987, a number of health ministers in African nations embraced the Bamako Initiative, a scheme promoted by the World Bank that advocated closing the health resource gap through user fees (Basilico et al. 2013: 89).

12. Scholars *have* examined changes to welfare provisions, including Bian and collaborators' (1997) investigation of changes to housing provision in Tianjin and Shanghai, Solinger's (1997, 1999) work on how the influx of migrant workers from rural China has changed urban workplace entitlements, and Mark Frazier's (2010) work on pension reform.

also now faces a dual burden of disease: infectious diseases (such as TB) remain a concern, while chronic conditions (e.g., diabetes and heart disease) have also been on the rise, particularly among China's aging population.

This book focuses on institutional changes that not only underlie the rise of migration but also resulted in the dissolution of basic-level public health and health-care infrastructure on which TB control depended. Studies have not systematically examined the effect of the rise and decline of the pervasive and intrusive work-unit system on health-care outcomes, particularly with respect to infectious disease. Certainly, no monograph has examined links between these institutional changes and the TB control challenges China now faces. This lack of scholarly attention is particularly surprising given the attention that has been paid to China with respect to other emerging infectious diseases, such as SARS and COVID-19, and China's debilitated public-health system following reform of basic health institutions.

Health in a Global City

Case selection

For this research, I focused on Shanghai because both historically and in the present day, Shanghai has been an industrial and financial leader, which makes it a prime candidate for an in-depth examination of the effect of institutional change on health outcomes. Mainland China's largest city has been important to global health, both historically and in the present day, because population growth, migration, travel, and trade allow for greater interconnectedness and opportunities for disease transmission. Likewise, in recent years, the reintroduction of market forces has led to growing inequality, including inequitable access to health care. Scholars have long acknowledged the importance of international travel and trade to the spread of infectious disease (McNeill 1977; Abu-Lughod 1989; Harrison 2012; Fang 2021). In recent decades, the globalization of trade has also been tied closely with neoliberalism, which emphasizes the primacy of market forces, including in the health sector. Saskia Sassen (1991, 2005) has emphasized the importance of global cities as critical nodes in the flow of information and capital, but Sassen's work has largely not addressed disease control.

Shanghai lies at a strategic geographic location, which has been important to its development. Shanghai, which means "on the sea," sits on the south bank of the Yangtze River as it empties into the East China Sea. The Yangtze's final tributary, the Huangpu River, cuts through the city and has always provided a convenient means of getting industrial goods to market, both within China and abroad. Following the First Opium War, in 1942, Shanghai was designated as a "treaty port," giving foreign powers access to its markets. Over the next century,

Table 0.2: Characteristics of dominant systems in Shanghai

	Pre-WUS	WUS (1950s–1990s)	Post-WUS
Global orientation	World city	China's industrial hub but globally isolated	Global city
Socioeconomic system	Capitalist	Communist	Socialism with market characteristics
Migration control system	Few regulations (except in the foreign concessions)	*Hukou* / residence permit system implemented in 1958	*Hukou* still largely in place but (arguably) declining in significance
Health access	Individual responsibility with provisions for key industries	Provided by workplace	Varies—largely fee for service based on a neoliberal model
PH system	Earliest state efforts	Mass mobilization	Professionalization
TB control	Pre-antibiotic era emphasis on social isolation in sanatoria	Active case finding with commitment to making antibiotics available in the workplace	Passive case finding with commitment to making antibiotics available for free

Figure 0.2: Shanghai's population growth

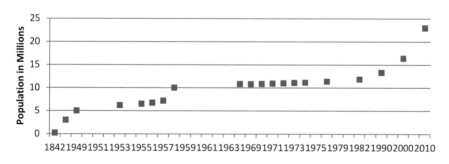

Source: Pre-1980 figures can be found in Ash 1981. Post-1980 figures are from census data.

16 *Tuberculosis Control and Institutional Change in Shanghai*

Shanghai's population and industry expanded rapidly. In 1928, Shanghai was a world city with a population around 3 million. It was China's leading port, industrial center, and financial capital. In the 1930s, the city's population continued to grow as peasants came to the city to escape the poverty of the countryside.

Shanghai was the country's most industrialized city from before 1949 through the 1980s. When the People's Republic of China was founded in 1949, Shanghai was designated as the administrative equivalent of a province. At the time, Shanghai's gross value of industrial output (GVIO) far exceeded that of China's two other independent municipalities with provincial distinction, Beijing and Tianjin, as well as all other provinces. Shanghai's GVIO was 21 percent of the national total in 1949, 16 percent of the national total in 1957, 17 percent of the national total in 1965, and 14 percent of the national total in 1977 (Howe 1981).

Shanghai was also China's most populous city throughout the mid-twentieth century. Between 1950 and 1958, Shanghai's population doubled from approximately 5 million to 10 million. Population growth in the 1950s occurred as a result of migration, a peacetime baby boom after years of war, and the 1958 annexation of rural counties needed to provide raw materials for industry and food for industrial workers. After 1958, Shanghai's population growth decelerated, then stagnated. Between the 1964 and 1982 censuses, Shanghai's population grew from 10.82 million to 11.86 million—with an average annual growth rate of only 0.5 percent (Zhu 2008). This population stabilization came about as a result of creation of the work-unit and *hukou* systems. Starting in 1958, the urban and rural populations were distinctly divided into nonagricultural and agricultural workers and issued residence permits designating them as either entitled to grain rations or not, and migration was strictly controlled. In the decade after Shanghai annexed 10 rural counties in 1958, much of the population there had agriculture residence permits, but rural industries were also important in some areas, which became the site of rapid industrial development in the 1980s. Most were eventually incorporated as urban districts during the 1990s.[13]

Since 1990, Shanghai has again experienced rapid population and economic growth. According to the 1990 census, Shanghai's population was only 13.34 million, but 20 years later it had grown to 23 million, mostly as a result of migration. Migrants have been attracted to Shanghai's booming economy, as the city

---

13. Highly industrialized Baoshan County, which is home to Bao Steel, was the first rural district to be incorporated, in 1988. In 1992, Jiading County became Jiading District, Chuansha County was incorporated as Pudong New District, and Shanghai County became Minhang District. Jinshan was incorporated in 1997, Songjiang in 1998, and Qingpu in 1999. Fengxian and Nanhui were incorporated in 2001, and Nanhui later became part of Pudong New District, in 2009. The only remaining rural county is Chongming Island. In recent years, some of the smaller urban districts merged with one another. For instance, Luwan District became part of Huangpu District in 2011. Likewise, Jiabei became part of Jing'an District in 2015.

Introduction 17

has been at the forefront of China's rapid economic growth in recent decades. Shanghai was one of the stops on Deng Xiaoping's Southern Tour, and his visit helped to solidify the notion that Pudong was to become a national showpiece for economic growth. The idea of Shanghai's return as an economic and trade center in the Asia Pacific was one that the State Council had proposed when it approved the 1986 Shanghai Municipal Master Plan. The State Council wanted Shanghai to play a leading role in reform and opening. It hoped to diversify Shanghai's economy beyond the traditional industrial base. The Pudong "new area," with Lujiazui as an international financial center, was to lead this regeneration (Hu and Chen 2019). Following a visit from Premier Li Peng, a Pudong Development Office opened in May 1990. In 1991, Pudong's first joint venture between a Chinese and an international company was established, and the Nanpu Bridge was completed, connecting areas of Shanghai on both sides of the Huangpu River. After Deng's visit in 1992, Pudong and Shanghai's growth accelerated.

Double-digit macroeconomic growth and rising inequality accompanied the shift toward capitalism. The 1990s saw increasing foreign investment and trade and China's successful bid to join the World Trade Organization (WTO). In 2020, Shanghai was truly a global city, home to the regional headquarters of more than 700 multinational corporations (Xinhua 2019). In the 1990s, the state moved away from dictating output targets and stopped allocating many goods and services. Per capita wages and household incomes have increased, but so has economic inequality, both nationally and within Shanghai. The trend of uneven development across China is illuminated by the United Nations Development Program's (UNDP's) subnational human development index (HDI), a composite measure of life expectancy, education, and per capita gross domestic product (GDP). Among mainland Chinese provinces, subnational HDI varies substantially, from a level rivaling that of low-income countries (in Tibet), to a level rivaling high income countries (in Beijing and Shanghai) (Permanyer and Smits 2018).

Growing mobility and inequality in the social realm has followed this growing economic inequality. China's Gini coefficient suggests that its levels of inequality now exceed those of the US and the UK (Jain-Chandar et al. 2016). Within Shanghai, tremendous wealth and poverty also exist side by side; while some have prospered, others have experienced exploitation and growing economic vulnerability. An additional change has been the return of class stratification. As China has moved toward the core of the global economic system, Chinese workers have experienced a profound loss of status (Goodman 2014). Capitalists are no longer shunned and have actually been accepted into the CCP. The clout of the emerging middle class has grown. Consumer goods and services are widely available to those who can afford them, but many cannot. Some flaunt their newfound wealth through conspicuous consumption—for example, zooming through the streets in luxury sports cars. Others who are attracted by the city's wealth are not so lucky and end up living in poverty.

TB was historically concentrated in urban areas, especially because of factors such as crowding, ambient air pollution, and industry. As China's largest and most industrialized city, with dense population and concentration of industry, Shanghai is a good case for looking at the roles of both TB in the workplace and the workplace in TB control. In the middle part of the twentieth century, TB was particularly prevalent among those who lived and worked in close quarters with little ventilation, such as the cotton mills, Shanghai's leading industry (Honig 1986). Crowded conditions led to increased opportunities for disease transmission, and Shanghai's TB incidence and mortality were extraordinarily high.

As China's wealthiest administrative region, Shanghai has also had more resources to provide to health care and public health services. Many of modern China's early disease control efforts, including efforts in TB control, were based there (Wong and Wu 1936). In contemporary China, the Center for Disease Control (CDC), modeled after the US CDC, was founded in Shanghai (Peng et al. 2003). Choosing Shanghai as my case has allowed me to examine implementation of TB control in a city that has, both historically and in the present day, been in a particularly advantageous position to implement new policies. With respect to TB control today, the municipality's health indicators—such as life expectancy and per capita health spending—suggest that it should be better poised to control the spread of TB than any other city, yet it still faces challenges.

Because the municipality includes both urban districts and rural counties (Figure 0.3), I was able to investigate institutional change in both urban and rural areas, which had very different types of economic and health-care systems. Just as Shanghai as a whole was the wealthiest and most developed area in China, its rural areas were in an advantageous position when compared to most of rural China. These advantages became most pronounced in the 1980s, when industry took off in the rural districts of Shanghai, along with other rural districts in China's coastal regions. I will note these important differences in my analysis.

Methods

This book draws heavily on two types of data: documents and interviews. I gathered the documents for both the historical and the current situation to understand the changing roles and effectiveness of the institutions of disease control. These documents were included in both published materials, such as newspapers, gazetteers, and yearbooks, and unpublished materials, such as records and reports from the archives of workplaces, hospitals, and schools. The published materials included those intended for both specialists in TB control and the general public. Many of these materials were published in the 1950s and 1960s

Figure 0.3: Map of Shanghai

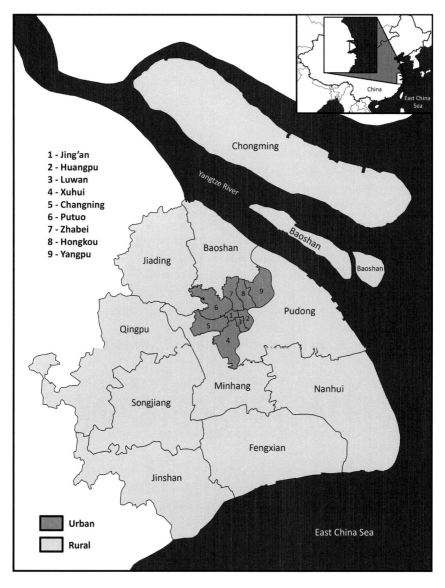

Source: Map by Clearview Geographic, LLC.

and emphasized disease control in the factory, school, or neighborhood. Finally, I gathered retrospective clinic reports from two district TB prevention and treatment clinics. These reports were crucial to understanding the division of responsibilities, interactions, support, and exchange of information among institutions active in the TB control network while the work-unit system was in place.

My research also involved embedding myself in two distinct and separate communities. First, I affiliated with a university, which helped me understand the work-unit system as it still exists. As a foreign student, I was entitled to use services at the school's hospital, and I received insurance to cover costs at higher-level facilities. I attended the public health programming on campus as a participant observer. Living in a dormitory would have allowed me further access to this community; however, I chose instead to live in a "new urban village" of laid-off workers near Suzhou Creek, Shanghai's light industrial hub, along which many of the former cotton factories once stood. This allowed me to interact daily with laid-off workers who now face challenges paying their children's school tuition and obtaining quality, affordable health care.

This new urban village was built in 1990 to house employees from several factories. When their factories closed around 2000, many were laid off and did not find stable reemployment. Lack of employment gave many of my neighbors time to volunteer for tasks assigned by the residents' committee, such as guarding the back gate or the bike shed. For my purposes, it meant I could always find laid-off workers with whom to discuss changes to China's health system. While I did not conduct formal, recorded interviews with any of my neighbors, I did take fieldnotes on my interactions. I spent an average of two hours per week talking with my neighbors between August 2010 and July 2011, about 100 hours total. They became my barometer for understanding the new challenges China's laid-off workers face.

I also conducted intensive interviews with 35 providers and 53 recipients of health care.[14] Providers of care included doctors and other health-care workers in workplaces, hospitals, clinics, and community health centers (CHCs). I recruited providers by going to hospitals, CHCs, and residents' committee offices and by using snowball sampling. I interviewed providers who worked under the work-unit system, providers who have worked under both systems, and providers who have worked since the work-unit system's decline to get insights into how tuberculosis control interventions have changed. Semistructured interviews included themes prompting discussion of health education campaigns, health monitoring, and access to treatment and care, both during the work-unit system and since its

---

14. The Johns Hopkins Homewood Institutional Review Board granted approval for this project in the summer of 2008 and approved renewals in 2009, 2010, 2011, and 2012.

Introduction 21

decline. Through these interviews, I was able to analyze both what institutions intended to provide and what they were actually able to provide.

In addition to providers of care, I interviewed care recipients. I especially targeted TB patients and members of their families. Forty-six of my 53 care recipients had experience as TB sufferers. These individuals were recruited through a respondent-driven method. I asked a few key informants who worked in the health system to give a card with my contact information to persons who have had family experience with TB. This card asked potential respondents to contact me if they would like to participate in the study. The questions I asked of care recipients were designed to historically compare TB control and the extent to which providers were successful in reaching the populace. As with the care providers, semi-structured interviews with recipients included themes prompting discussion of health education campaigns, case finding, and access to treatment and care both during the work-unit system and since its decline. The interview protocol included probes to seek information about how access issues affected health and illness behavior both during the work-unit system and since its transformation. Given that my sample was respondent driven, a number of younger TB patients also contacted me to discuss their illness experience. Their experiences provide a fuller picture of the spectrum of health-care coverage that is available in contemporary China.

Structure of the Book

This book is divided chronologically into seven chapters and three parts. Part I examines disease control in Shanghai before 1949. Chapter 1 investigates the colonial state's tardiness in addressing TB between 1911 and 1927, both because other diseases were more acute and because controlling TB would have entailed improving social conditions for the local population. The chapter examines the difficult trade-off leaders have to make when considering whether to prioritize disease control or economic growth. Chapter 2 turns to 1928–1949, when the GMD state became committed to strengthening the nation. Despite best intentions and some cooperation between governmental and nongovernmental actors, TB prevention, in particular, was not targeted to members of the population who lived and worked under conditions that made them particularly susceptible. War interrupted some TB prevention efforts, but nonprofit actors attempted to make beds more widely available, even during the 1937–1945 Japanese Occupation. Efforts became even more widespread in the postwar years. The section concludes that the foundation upon which the Communists would build public health work was set before 1949.

Part II examines Shanghai between 1950 and 1992. Chapter 3 focuses on the 1950–1957 creation of the work-unit system; Chapter 4 focuses on urban disease control at the 1958–1992 height of the urban work-unit system; and Chapter 5 focuses on disease control in Shanghai's rural counties. Chapter 3 introduces the model of the new health image the state aimed to create. In the 1950s, the workplace-based TB control program was developed and began to be scaled up to make scientific and public health advances available to the masses. While the model was never fully realized, Shanghai still saw dramatic declines in TB mortality and morbidity.

Chapter 4 covers 1958 to 1992, a period during which maturation of the work-unit system, the urban health system, and the urban TB control network occurred. The types of care individuals received in different types of enterprises varied; however, almost all urban residents had basic health coverage. During these decades, personnel from district prevention and treatment clinics worked closely with workplace doctors to identify TB sufferers and monitor their care. Particularly during the 1980s, the municipal government also relied on cooperation between residents' committees and public health nurses to reach members of the population who might not have been served in their work units. Coverage was never complete, but the chapter demonstrates that these collective efforts contributed to declining TB.

Chapter 5 turns to the case of Shanghai's rural counties to examine how the workplace-based cooperative medical system developed and facilitated TB control. This system was particularly effective in delivering low-cost preventive health care and controlling costs from the 1960s to the 1980s. The chapter argues that the rural health system remained largely intact in rural Shanghai throughout the 1980s, due in large part to financial support from township and village enterprises, but this finding is unlikely to be generalizable to the rest of China, because the number of township and village enterprise (TVEs) in Shanghai exceeded that of other areas.

Part III examines the initial deleterious effects of China's turn toward the market on the medical and public health systems after 1992. Chapter 6 investigates the major demographic and economic changes dominated the 1990s: privatization, the shedding of welfare responsibilities by employers, a shift to less permanent employment and the rise of migration. The 1990s also saw a restructuring of the health and TB control systems—leading to the variation in coverage that has contributed to new challenges in TB control. Indeed, while China made an incomplete leap forward in health in the middle part of the twentieth century, this work concludes that maintenance of health-care and public health infrastructure is crucial to making medical advances available, both for controlling TB as well as emerging diseases, such as COVID-19.

Part I

Republican Era, 1911–1949

1

Tuberculosis and the Quest for Modernity in Shanghai, 1911–1927

On March 20, 1914, the Annual Meeting of the Ratepayers of Shanghai's International Settlement voted down a special resolution to found a tuberculosis hospital. During the meeting, persons in favor of the resolution spoke of the urgent need for a benevolent institution to treat a disease "found very largely among the poorer population of Shanghai" ("Resolution VII" 1914: 97). After the resolution had already been seconded, Dr. H. C. Patrick delivered a screed, raising objections on several points, including the unreliability of TB diagnoses and mortality statistics—he believed many so-called TB cases were actually cases of malnutrition. He also questioned the location of the intended structure, which went against the previous plan to build on the site of the Municipal Isolation Hospital. The 465 ratepayers in attendance chuckled at his remarks on ambiguous statements regarding the danger of spitting and his insistence that effort not be wasted on educating cases "of a hopeless nature." Perhaps most damning was Dr. Patrick's claim that the hospital would likely be "little better than a home for those dying of tuberculosis" ("Tuberculosis Hospital" 1915: 94). While this comment should have underscored the need for such a hospital, it led to defeat of the resolution, which ultimately delayed the hospital by five years and dealt a blow to controlling the most widespread and deadly disease in Shanghai. The debate also encapsulates the wider debates raging over the "TB Question" at the beginning of the twentieth century, both in Shanghai and globally. How effective was it to isolate a few cases, when tuberculosis was so widespread?

The TB Question was the problem of how to control infectious disease that tracks largely on socioeconomic lines (LaMotte 1908). Breaking the chain of infection by isolating TB sufferers was certainly part of the solution to preventing future infections, but it would not address the underlying conditions that made the poor vulnerable to TB—overcrowded housing and exploitative labor conditions. Many of Shanghai's ratepayers were born abroad and maintained close personal and financial connections to their overseas homes, so they were likely aware of the discussion happening on the international stage, from New York, to London, to Berlin (Strachan 1933; Bryder 1988; Teller 1988; Sanitize and Shengelia 2015). Thus, Shanghai's civic leaders and social reformers—both Chinese and international—grappled with many of the same issues being explored elsewhere around the globe. Truly controlling TB would have meant undertaking quality-of-life interventions, which were generally anathema to profit, a pressing concern for many of the International Settlement's ratepayers. This chapter examines why TB control was not prioritized during the first 17 years of the Republic of China, despite growing attention to TB control globally, and growing attention to infectious disease control in Shanghai and China more generally. At the crux of the ratepayers' debate was an important question: If industrialization and urbanization result in conditions conducive to spreading TB, was curtailing these processes the solution for stopping TB? Few business or government leaders would advocate for slower economic growth. As today's leaders have had to make tough decisions regarding the trade-offs between curtailing the economy and controlling COVID-19, early twentieth-century reformers around the world faced difficult decisions regarding interventions with respect to TB.

Controlling infectious disease, the rise of public health, and accommodation of Western medicine have closely aligned with China's quest for modernity (Rogaski 2004; Bu 2009, 2017; Lei 2014; Andrews 2014, 2015; N. E. Barnes 2018; Baum 2018; Nakajima 2018; Brazelton 2019b). Despite similar overlaps between the TB and modernization movements, China's formal tuberculosis movement began only in 1933, decades later than in other places around the globe. Yet, as this chapter demonstrates, in the 1910s Shanghai's leaders were already debating two public health recommendations arising in conjunction with the global anti-TB movement: isolating disease sufferers and regulating labor. Several governments around the globe supported the sanatorium movement or labor laws to help curb TB. Indeed, health is a way that nations might gain legitimacy in the eyes of their own citizens, or at least other nations, as China did during the Manchurian plague of 1910–1911. Given the relative instability throughout China's territories under the Warlord period of the 1910s, and the First World War, it is unsurprising that Shanghai was unable to maintain consistent focus on public health, but this chapter will highlight several important areas of cooperation. Lessons from the Manchurian plague will be discussed, including the impetus toward collaboration between health organizations, and between government actors and health organizations.

This chapter demonstrates that those who wanted to control TB faced difficult choices regarding where to aim their interventions. Should they simply provide a technical solution in the form of isolation facilities? Could efforts really be effective without attention to the socioeconomic and underlying determinants of health? The search for answers to these questions in China was similar to the quest TB control reformers undertook in other places around the globe, and yet, Shanghai's governments largely did not tackle TB until the 1920s. Scholars such as Ruth Rogaski have characterized Shanghai during this time as "hypercolonial," because it was divided among multiple imperial powers (2004: 11). The city had the Chinese City, as well as two concessions, where foreigners had extraterritorial rights: the French Concession, and a British-dominated International Settlement. The Chinese City did not have a health department until 1926, so health data from that section of the city are only fragmentary (Jackson 2017; Nakajima 2018). Consequently, the chapter draws largely on data collected by the International Settlement's health department because they were the most comprehensive data available; however, as will be discussed, they were nevertheless far from complete. The data serve as a blurry snapshot of conditions in a place where some interventions were made to control health behaviors.

Recent scholarship has revisited the International Settlement's governing body, the Shanghai Municipal Council (SMC), and demonstrated its importance in shaping modern Shanghai (Jackson 2017).The SMC was largely concerned with promoting economics and trade, but a health department was also founded in 1898. The existence of this department signaled that health was a nominal concern, and health became a point of contention between the colonizer and the colonized, as has been the case in many colonial settings (Arnold 1991; Anderson 1995; Rogaski 2004, Furth 2011; Lei 2014; Packard 2016; Jackson 2017). In the International Settlement, the choice about whether to prioritize health or the economy was originally made in favor of the economy: support for health was paltry.[1] The SMC's budget was already very lean, because of an acute aversion to taxation prior to 1928.[2] The health department's budget paled in comparison to those of the police department and the public works department. The health department's apportionment did increase over the decades, but in 1930, 43 percent of the municipal budget went to policing, 30 percent to public works, and a meager 7 percent sliver to health (Jackson 2012: 214). Certainly, both the police and public works departments provided services to the health department—police provided security, and public works maintained infrastructure, including hospitals—but the municipal coffers did not have much money to support public health interventions, especially for Chinese residents. However, as this chapter illustrates, the SMC's concern about disease control and

---

1. The SMC Health Department had only two leaders during the period covered in this chapter. Arthur Stanley led the department from its founding until 1921. Starting in the spring of 1921, Noel Davis became acting commissioner of public health and then led the department from 1922 to 1930. From 1930 to 1943, J. H. Jordan led the department.
2. In 1928, after Chinese councillors were finally brought into the SMC's decision-making process, attention to the health of Chinese residents increased.

health of Chinese residents eventually grew, due to the realization that there was no bubble protecting foreign residents.

The Rise of Anti-TB Organizations Globally

Perhaps more than any other disease, tuberculosis has closely aligned with the quest for modernization in nations throughout the globe. Even before Robert Koch's 1882 discovery of the tuberculosis bacillus, social reformers at various locations recognized a relationship between tuberculosis and industrialization. Industrialization demanded labor, which factory owners hoped to extract as cheaply as possible. This led to low wages, often accompanied by long hours and unsafe working conditions, which made workers vulnerable by compromising their immune systems and exposing them to disease outbreaks in the factory. Workers were packed, often side by side, along assembly lines in enclosed spaces with little ventilation. At the end of their shift, they carried the disease home to their dormitories and other crowded urban spaces where they lived (Honig 1986; Johnston 1995). Consequently, regulating labor became a concern. Koch's discovery catalyzed efforts to implement several quality-of-life and public health interventions to control tuberculosis. Until antibiotics were discovered, manufactured and widely distributed, a number of general social interventions and public health measures were undertaken to control infectious disease. Many locations founded anti-tuberculosis leagues and associations, which became models for future disease control efforts.[3] Generally, these organizations were nonprofits; however, many received state funding, and some were state organizations. All aimed to influence policy.

As one example, in the United States, leading health reformers founded the National Tuberculosis Association (NTA) in 1904 to coordinate TB control efforts, both nationally and internationally.[4] This nonprofit organization's objectives included disseminating knowledge—both to the public and to government health organizations (Strachan 1933; Perkins 1954; Teller 1988). The NTA

---

3. As Bryder (1988) notes, anti-TB associations were established in France in 1891, Pennsylvania in 1892, Germany in 1895, Belgium and Britain in 1898, Italy and Portugal in 1899, Canada in 1900, Australia (New South Wales and Victoria) and Denmark in 1901, Sweden and the United States in 1904, Japan in 1908, and Norway and Russia in 1909 (15–16). Guttiérrez (2017) examines efforts in Cuba, where the League against TB in Cuba was formally established in 1901. Likewise, Morelo-Mesa (2010) notes that Spanish and Catalonian organizations to fight TB were set up in Madrid and Barcelona in 1903; the Spanish Anti-TB Association later formed the base for a state anti-TB organization (177).

4. Those leaders included William Welch (1850–1934) and William Osler (1849–1919), founders of the Johns Hopkins Hospital; Edward Livingston Trudeau (1848–1915), founder of the sanatorium Saranac Lake; and S. A. Knopf (1857–1940), a German American physician who specialized in TB treatment.

researched TB from both a medical and social perspective, and it standardized work of local and state TB agencies (Strachan 1933; Perkins 1954). Through close cooperation with state institutions, it often blurred the boundaries between official and voluntary organizations (Perkins 1954). The voluntary organizations coordinated with the state on education campaigns, which used posters, slogans, exhibits, slide shows, and films to improve knowledge (Teller 1988). Moreover, the association also cooperated with other organizations internationally.

International anti-TB organizations also grappled with quality-of-life debates, similar to those debated at the Shanghai ratepayers meeting in March 1914. In the United States, the social determinants of health, in particular economic conditions of the poor and working classes, were one of the biggest concerns of the NTA. During the Progressive Era, writers and other social reformers attempted to raise awareness of social conditions for the purpose of catalyzing social change. For example, photojournalist and social reformer Jacob Riis published pictures highlighting the deplorable conditions in New York's tenements, many of which were occupied by recent European immigrants (1890). Riis made a direct connection between living conditions and the spread of infectious disease in his work on typhus and police boarding houses (1893). TB was very personal for Riis because six of his brothers had died of it, and in 1907, he published an article on the use of Christmas seals in his native Denmark, which inspired the first Christmas Seal campaign in America (1907; Christensen 1968). Likewise, Upton Sinclair published his muckraking novel, *The Jungle*, which illuminated Chicago's deplorable factory conditions in 1906, just after the NTA was founded. In *The Jungle*, an elderly Lithuanian immigrant, Anatas, loses his toes because of chemical exposure at work and dies of an unnamed disease whose symptoms, which included coughing blood and weight loss, were characteristic of TB. This character was fictional but was based on the reality of exploitative labor and crowded living conditions among immigrants. The NTA built upon the momentum of the Progressive Era, taking it upon itself to "solve such problems as malnutrition, substandard housing, and inadequate welfare assistance programs" (Perkins 1954: 515).

In terms of "treatment," prior to the discovery of effective antibiotics, the internationally accepted remedy was rest and fresh air. This "treatment" was often combined with the public health "solution" of isolating sick individuals, which resulted in their removal from their communities, particularly if they lived in crowded urban areas. Edward Livingston Trudeau spearheaded the US sanatorium movement. While unsuccessfully nursing his brother back to health, Trudeau contracted TB and recovered by leaving New York City and adopting an outdoor lifestyle in the Adirondack Mountains. Following his recovery, he encouraged others to take up this "cure" and founded a sanatorium at Saranac Lake, New York, in 1885. Although some scholars have argued that this sanatorium's primary contribution was housing and feeding charity cases, separation from the community was also key to interrupting transmission (Mera 1935; Teller 1988).

The US sanatorium movement gained steam with the completion of the transcontinental railway in 1869. Sheila Rothman's work investigates how seeking a cure for tuberculosis compelled thousands of Americans to move to the West by wagon train and rail. Attracted to sunlight and wide open spaces, they settled in Colorado Springs, Albuquerque, and Pasadena, among other places. While this "cure" often did not work, this did not stop the proliferation of businesses who desired to make money from health seekers, including real estate investors, sanatoria with sun porches, and a host of businesses to service them (Mera 1935; Rothman 1994).

The US efforts were inspired, in part, by an equally vibrant sanatorium movement in Europe. Many European leaders, physicians, and members of the public had accepted the notion that some conditions were more favorable to healing than others. Both general health retreats, known as sanitaria, and institutions specifically for treating TB, sanatoria, were set up at favorable locations throughout the continent, such as the Swiss Alps.[5] Hermann Brehmer established Europe's first *Kurhaus* (sanatorium) in 1862. It had 40 beds initially and had expanded to 100 beds at the time Koch discovered the TB bacillus in 1882 (Daniel 2011; Eylers 2014). When the US NTA was founded 1904, Brehmer's sanatorium was the largest facility in the world, with 300 beds. As in the United States, both sanitaria and sanatoria could be thriving businesses, but efforts to found institutions for charity cases also existed, both to protect the general public and to remove the sick from the conditions prompting their ill health.

In China, the Anti-TB organization that would eventually be founded in 1933 would adopt many of the characteristics and tactics of the international TB movements, such as the US NTA. For instance, as the next chapter illustrates, the Chinese organization likewise blurred boundaries between state and social organizations. It also relied heavily on media, such as posters, slogans, exhibits, slide shows, and films. The National Anti-Tuberculosis Association of China became the longest-serving single-disease-focused organization in China, but by the time of its founding, other countries had shifted away from TB control as a major priority, as geopolitical entanglements took center stage (D. S. Barnes 1995: 18).

---

5. Rothman claims that the nineteenth century Western public would have known the distinction between sanitaria and sanatoria (1994: 157); however, English language reports from organizations in Shanghai use the terms interchangeably. To avoid confusion, I update the term to "sanatorium," when the institution in question is devoted to TB treatment.

In 1910s Shanghai, the idea of moving infectious individuals from crowded areas to the countryside was already accepted by Chinese elites, Western missionary doctors, and colonial governments. However, widespread acceptance does not mean that the will existed to carry it out or that it had widespread public support. In fact, as the opening vignette illustrates, the first efforts to found a designated TB sanatorium in Shanghai had difficulty getting off the ground. After investigating the example of China's response to the Manchurian plague as a way the nation reasserted autonomy regarding health, this chapter will turn more directly to the largely unsuccessful TB control efforts in Shanghai.

The Manchurian Plague as the Catalyst for Public Health Work in China

TB was not the only respiratory disease that played an important part in China's medical modernization. The 1910–1911 pneumonic plague, which killed 60,000 people in Manchuria, has been widely studied as a critical event leading to the rise of public health in China (Andrews 2011, 2014; Summers 2012; Lynteris 2013; Lei 2014; Hanson 2017; Soon 2020). Because it has been studied in detail elsewhere, this section will provide only the briefest outline of the event itself, focusing instead on the lessons and cooperative organizations arising from that experience. In the years following the plague, various organizations, both public and private, stepped up to control infectious disease, an area that China identified as a way of strengthening its population and demonstrating its power on an international stage.

The extremely acute and deadly pneumonic plague appeared along the Manchurian border with Russia in October 1910. Human-animal contact is believed to have been the source of the outbreak. Specifically, tarbagans, a type of Manchurian marmots, were overhunted for their pelts, and hunters became infected (Lynteris 2013). By November 1910, Fujiadian, a district where many Chinese laborers resided just beyond the official limits of the multicultural city of Harbin, became the epicenter of the outbreak (Gamsa 2006). Over the next six months, the plague spread southward along the railway (Summers 2012; Lynteris 2013; Hanson 2017). In response to this fast-acting and deadly pathogen, the Chinese government enlisted the services of a Cambridge-trained overseas Chinese physician from Penang, Wu Liande (Wu Lien-teh, 伍连德). Wu implemented infection control protocols, such as social distancing and masking, which curbed the infection. Following these successes, the Chinese government amplified its voice as an actor on the stage of international health by convening a conference to discuss lessons from its pneumonic plague intervention (Lei 2014; Lynteris 2018; Brazelton 2020; Soon and Chong 2020).

Several broad lessons arose from China's experience with the pneumonic plague, such as the need for international cooperation in preventing epidemics, isolation as an intervention to halt the spread of communicable diseases, and quick and decisive state response to outbreaks. Tuberculosis control in Shanghai during this era benefited from these first two lessons, but not the final one. Shanghai saw some attempts at international cooperation in disease control. Likewise, in keeping with international protocols, isolation was recognized as one of the important disease control mechanisms. However, despite TB being the most widespread disease, governments in Shanghai did not take swift and decisive action. Instead, they stalled. Indeed, tuberculosis is not as acute or as deadly as the pneumonic plague, so lack of swift action did not have the deleterious effects that hesitation would have with the plague. Before turning to why the state did not take swift and decisive action against TB, the rest of this section discusses the cooperation that arose between public health organizations that were active in China in the decades after its success with plague control.

In the decades following the Manchurian plague, numerous organizations capitalized on the recognized need for international cooperation in preventing epidemics. These entities included multilateral organizations (such as the League of Nations Health Organization), international organizations (such as the Rockefeller Foundation), both national and local government organizations (such as the Central Epidemic Prevention Bureau and the SMC Health Department) and private and nonprofit associations (such as the YMCA and China Medical Missionary Association). Recent years have also seen growing interest in the League of Nations Health Organization, but that organization was not founded until 1924, and it was largely not active in China until after 1928 (Borowy 2009; Jackson 2017; Brazelton 2019b). As with TB control, the rise of PH more generally has been tied to the process of modernization, and it is equally contested. With the rise of more modern factories, there was a need for healthier workers, and productivity became closely tied with public health. As scholars have argued, worldwide thinking about health of the poorer classes shifted from a moral to an economic standpoint (D. S. Barnes 1995; Andrews 2011, 2015). Both the moral and economic approaches to the poor have social control as their aim; however, the economic approach recognizes wider culpability and responsibility of the wealthier classes in creating conditions to uplift the poor. This involved widening the lens of public health to include social conditions. If moral approbation was not the cause of ill health, disease sufferers need not be punished. Policy implications followed this shifting view of public health. Thus, in the 1910s, China also saw a shift from the draconian PH measures aimed at controlling plague to more publicity-based community health interventions (Jackson 2017: 201). Shanghai had more resources than did other Chinese cites, but finding the resources to support health and public health became a contested space. The SMC devoted only a sliver of its budget to health, meaning that many health interventions were run by nonprofits. Multiple organizations conflicted over and collaborated on public health interventions.

Among the international organizations most active in China was the Rockefeller Foundation's China Medical Board (CMB) and the League of Nations Health Organization (LNHO). The CMB was established in 1914 and counted founding the Peking Union Medical College (PUMC) among its early accomplishments. However the CMB's early leaders came to the conclusion that the organization itself should not get involved in widescale public health work for several reasons. Among them, the CMB noted that confidence in Western medicine was not widespread in China, nor did China have a sufficient number of trained health personnel. The PUMC was founded as a response to this latter point. Perhaps most importantly, the CMB viewed public health as a government responsibility (Lei 2014). While many of the PH interventions undertaken by the Rockefeller Foundation were directed toward rural areas, some were also relevant to urban areas. In particular, the Rockefeller Foundation's mission was intimately tied to capitalism: it was funded by capitalists and aimed to promote healthy urban workers (Bu 2009).

National-level organizations were too varied to survey here but included organizations aimed at specific diseases (such as the Northern Manchurian Plague Prevention Service), controlling communicable disease outbreaks more generally (such as the Central Epidemic Prevention Bureau), and controversial attempts to promote Western medicine in China (such as by the China Medical Association). The China Medical Association (CMA) was established in 1915 and held its first national conference in Shanghai in 1916. Given its name, one might assume it was an organization of Chinese professionals, but foreign doctors originally comprised the vast majority of its members. The number of Western-trained Chinese nationals who joined the organization increased after its founding, but in 1929, only 100 of its 700 members were Chinese. While this organization's goals were largely dedicated to scientific research and promoting Western medicine—it published the *China Medical Journal*—public health was also part of its mission. Following its first annual meeting, one of the five recommendations to the government focused on control of tuberculosis (and venereal disease) (Wong and Wu 1936: 771–72).

In Shanghai, several organizations cooperated with respect to health education, including both public and private organizations. While cooperation was initially limited during the 1910s, it became closer in the early 1920s. As an example of early public-private cooperation, the SMC's branch health offices worked closely with private organizations on educational and immunization campaigns. In a similar vein, in 1916, the CMA, Chinese Medical Missionary Association (CMMA), and the Young Men's Christian Association (YMCA) cooperated to form the Joint Council on Health Education (Bu 2009; Jackson 2017: 172). Likewise, in August 1920, the SMC health officer reported that the Joint Council on Health Education, the CMMA, and the CMA, were working together to develop the Municipal Health Office's notices and booklets on prevention of the diseases prevalent in China (Stanley 1920a: 324). The report also praised the YMCA for educating people throughout China on the fundamentals of sanitation through lantern slide demonstrations and open-air lectures. This work would continue in the upcoming years. The January 1921 *Health Officer's Report (HOR)* also noted that talks were being given at branch health offices, and in 1924 the CMMA, the China Christian Educational Association, the YMCA, and the Young Women's Christian Association Nurses Association convened a Conference on School Health (Stanley 1921: 47; Wong and Wu 1936: 673). All of these interventions signaled growing attention to health; however, as will be discussed in the next section, to truly address TB, officials would have to address problems related to socioeconomic conditions, but not many were committed to this.

Disease Control in a Hypercolonial City

As a disease that killed slowly, rather than quickly, TB did not require the same swift and decisive action as did the Manchurian plague. That said, tuberculosis deserved attention because it was the single most deadly disease in early twentieth-century China. Unfortunately, comprehensive statistics regarding disease prevalence throughout the nation were not taken until the mid-1920s. The Association for the Advancement of Public Health conducted the first comprehensive census of vital statistics in China from September 1925 to February 1926 at health stations in northern China. According to their findings with respect to 10 infectious diseases, pulmonary tuberculosis caused the highest number of deaths. The TB mortality rate of 445.5 per 100,000 was five times that of England (Bowers 1974). More conservative estimates of 300–350 per 100,000 were still much higher than the TB mortality rates of 114 in the United States and 215 in Japan during that time (Yip 1995).

More comprehensive statistics were collected in parts of Shanghai starting at an earlier date; however, Shanghai's demography remained a "puzzle with missing pieces" (Henriot 2016: 40). Over the four and a half decades that it was active (1898–1943), the SMC Health Department monitored disease outbreaks and kept records of causes of death, to the extent that it was known. As Foucault has argued, counting and gaining statistics about bodies is an act of governmentality of the state onto the population. Tong Lam has examined the production of social facts in the creation of a new social order under the hypercolonial environment that was early twentieth-century China (2011: 14). SMC leaders used the

Tuberculosis and the Quest for Modernity

health statistics to justify their policies pertaining not just to foreigners but also to the "native" population of the foreign concessions. In fact, most residents of the International Settlement were Chinese, so the SMC also collected data on these Chinese residents. While health officials were originally only concerned about the health of Chinese residents insofar as they were a potential source of infection, interventions against Chinese citizens were also made by the SMC. These policies were as noninvasive as efforts to widely administer smallpox vaccines and as invasive as demolishing homes found to be out of compliance with plague-prevention recommendations.

Starting in 1908, the Shanghai Municipal Council began reporting infectious disease cases and deaths among foreigners and deaths among Chinese weekly in the *Shanghai Municipal Gazette*; however, these data grossly undercount disease incidence and death among Chinese residents. On any given day, dozens of Chinese corpses were discarded throughout the city (including mostly children under five), and the cause of death for these individuals was not recorded (Henriot 2009, 2016). Diseases listed in *Health Officer's Report* varied somewhat from year to year. In addition to tuberculosis, the notifiable diseases initially included smallpox, cholera, typhoid fever, diphtheria, scarlet fever, and plague. Dysentery, measles, paratyphoid, cerebrospinal fever, and influenza were also sometimes added to the list.[6] TB was consistently the deadliest disease on an annual basis, but commentary in most monthly public health reports focused on more acute diseases, which led to quicker deaths. Thus, the diseases that Shanghai's leaders were most concerned about were the same ones that were prevalent in other ports—both along China's coast and inland along the Yangtze (Benedict 1996; Rogaski 2004; Hanson 2017). To some extent, they were also the diseases prevalent in other colonial ports in South Asia (Arnold 1991).

Depending on the season, diseases other than TB were prevalent or saw flare-ups. For instance, some winter reports discuss respiratory diseases, such as measles and influenza; spring reports discuss scarlet fever; and summer reports discuss gastrointestinal illnesses, including cholera and dysentery. The outbreaks that occurred in the 1910s are well documented in the monthly reports. As an example, an outbreak of measles started in November 1911 and peaked in early 1912, with 156 deaths among Chinese during the month of March 1912 (Stanley 1912: 123). Other notable outbreaks included the 142 deaths from scarlet fever among Chinese citizens in April 1917 (Stanley 1917: 153). Like many places

---

6. In 1909–1914, the seven notifiable diseases were smallpox, cholera, typhoid fever, diphtheria, scarlet fever, tuberculosis, and plague. By 1915, dysentery was sometimes added to the list; it tended to be reported only on a monthly, rather than a weekly, basis. After 1917, measles and paratyphoid fever were sometimes reported, as well. Cerebrospinal fever and influenza were sometimes reported starting in 1919. (Statistics for beriberi was also sometimes reported, but it is vitamin deficiency rather than an infectious disease.)

around the globe, Shanghai saw deaths from the "Spanish flu" and started including them in its monthly reports as a result. In March 1919, an influenza outbreak killed 342 Chinese and 23 foreigners, prompting encouragement of face mask usage (Stanley 1919a: 146).[7] As the *Health Officer's Reports* for 1920 and 1921 note, the month of May was often a welcome reprieve between the winter onslaught of respiratory diseases and the summer spike in food-borne illnesses.

Plague was among the most worrisome diseases because of it is acute and deadly, and many health department reports focus on its control. Plague-infected rodents were first discovered in Shanghai in 1908, and the ever-present fear of outbreak prompted the SMC Health Department to monitor the situation and take measures to eliminate rats. For instance, according to the March 1909 *Health Officer's Report*, plague had not made headway in the Eastern, Western, or Central Districts, but the number of plague-infected rats in the Northern District had increased. Plague had also been detected in Zhabei District, on the settlement's border, so dead rats were examined in municipal labs (Stanley 1909: 124). At the household level, citizens were encouraged to take several measures to eliminate plague: keeping cats, poisoning or trapping and burning rats, properly storing food and disposing of refuse, and covering crawlspaces and drains to prevent rodents' entry. Despite these efforts, dozens of plague-infected rats were found each year prior to 1916, and a handful of human cases of bubonic plague were found in several years. After 1916, there was still the possibility of plague arriving by rail or ship, but efforts started to pay off.

Table 1.1: Annual incidence of plague

	1908	1909	1910	1911	1912	1913	1914	1915	1916	1917	1918	1919
Infected rats	49	187	249	138	95	122	186	76	6	0	0	0
Human cases	0	0	6	0	18	10	26	1	0	0	0	0

Source: *Annual Report of the Shanghai Municipal Council*, 1919.

Cholera was likewise feared in treaty ports throughout China, because of its explosive infectiousness and deadly nature. In an attempt to control frequent cholera outbreaks, Shanghai built China's first waterworks to pipe water to some residents of the International Settlement in the 1880s (MacPherson 1987). However, this does not mean that health department recommendations regarding

---

7. While *Health Officer's Reports* were published in most months, in 1918, none were issued between April and December, so the monthly death count for Spanish flu (and TB) are not readily available.

cholera were readily embraced by all local residents even three decades later. There had been a severe cholera epidemic in September 1907 and lesser epidemics in 1909–1910 and 1912, but vigilance managed to stave off severe epidemics for most of the decade. Outbreaks prompted interventions aimed at the poor and the working poor, including notices regarding food sanitation and licensing of food vendors. However, the SMC Health Department encountered both active and passive resistance by the urban poor. Interventions included issuing bilingual notices reminding residents to sterilize food through cooking or boiling, but persons who could not read may not have paid attention to or fully grasped the content of these notices. Some residents may have ignored the notices, but they could not escape feeling the effect of licensing. The 1912 outbreak intensified pressure toward licensing food sellers. The SMC's 1912 *Annual Report* noted the resulting "objection to interfering with the old customs of the wharf" (SMC 1913: 62A). The health department aimed to curtail itinerant hawkers' practice of selling "fly-infected" food to coolies, but licensing entailed controversial fees. This issue continued to simmer for years, but measures seemed to be working until late in the decade. Resistance was most clearly felt when a mob attacked the branch health offices (BHOs) at the end of April 1918. The mob was believed to be hawkers protesting a hike in licensure fees (Stanley 1918b: 166–67). The 1918 protests and the cholera outbreak in 1919—which killed 222 Chinese and 10 foreigners in the month of August—prompted reminders on how to use boiled water to sterilize produce, such as grapes and strawberries (Stanley 1919b: 313, 1920c; SMC 1920). But clearly these measures would not have been available to the urban poor, who often lacked access to piped water and had limited facilities for boiling it.

In addition to seasonal outbreaks and extremely acute infections, the SMC Health Department focused on dissemination of known preventive remedies. For instance, one of the health department's early tasks was administering smallpox vaccines. By 1912, sixteen subdistrict health stations had been created, each of which served approximately 30,000 residents (SMC 1913). These BHOs were responsible for sanitation and immunizations within the subdistrict. The 1912 SMC *Annual Report* noted that when "smallpox has been stamped out by bringing free vaccination almost to the doors of all the people, it will be possible to attack the greatest of all modern health problems, the prevention of tuberculosis" (SMC 1913: 62A). Paving the way for smallpox eradication, BHOs provided thousands of free vaccinations to Chinese residents each year. By 1919, a total of 144,000 doses had been administered, and the numbers increased in the following decade (SMC 1920). During the winter of 1920–1921 alone, a total of 14,400 smallpox vaccinations were given (N. Davis 1921: 231). As education on vaccination continued, the number administered by the BHOs more than doubled to 30,000 in 1922 (N. Davis 1923: 16). Despite these efforts, smallpox flare-ups occurred in Shanghai. TB could not be the focus of similar inoculation efforts because the BCG vaccine was not proven effective until the early 1920s and certified by the League of Nations in 1928.

Aside from seasonal flare-ups and acute outbreaks, tuberculosis was the leading cause of death in almost all months throughout Shanghai the 1910s and 1920s. Deaths among Chinese and diagnosed cases among foreigners were reported on a weekly basis, and deaths among foreigners and Chinese were reported on a monthly basis. In most weeks between 1911 and 1920, zero new cases were reported among foreigners, and there were generally 10–25 deaths among Chinese. On a monthly basis, there were 10 or fewer deaths from TB among foreigners in almost all months and several dozen deaths among Chinese every month.[8] For the decade, monthly deaths among Chinese citizens ranged from 35 in February 1911, to 124 in April 1918. The weekly high for this period was 39 known deaths from TB among Chinese for the week ending on September 3, 1916. There was a marked increase in the weekly and monthly numbers as the decade progressed, suggesting either that conditions deteriorated or that the figures from the early part of the 1910s reflected statistical undercounting, or perhaps a bit of both. Given the consistently high deaths from TB, there was surprisingly little attention paid to it in the Monthly *Health Officer's Reports* and correspondence in the Shanghai Municipal Archives, but there is some. In particular, two times exhibited a good bit of attention to TB: 1913–1915 and 1921–1922, both of which will be described below.

The Struggle for a Municipal Sanatorium, 1913–1919

The approach that officials in Shanghai hoped to take against TB was heavily influenced by recommendations of tuberculosis associations around the globe, including the sanatorium movement. Shanghai needed more places to isolate TB sufferers, but where to do so and what resources could be used for this purpose were under debate. Before the world was fully enmeshed in World War I, there was much discussion about the need for the Municipal Council Sanatorium. Between 1913 and 1915, the issue of trying to found such a hospital was hotly debated between the SMC secretary, health officers, and several other concerned parties, including doctors and charitable organizations. The facility finally received support from the SMC ratepayers in March 2015, one year after it was originally voted down. It then took more than four years to build and fully staff it, in part because of the war.

---

8. In the 1910s, monthly statistics were almost always published in the *Health Officer's Reports*. Very few months had more than 10 deaths from TB among foreigners.

Correspondence on the issue began on April 30, 1913, when the governors of the Shanghai General Hospital implored the SMC Health Department to find a suitable location for treatment of TB sufferers: "Treatment of patients with TB lung disease is most undesirable under the same roof as general hospital patients" (SMA U1-16-617). The words "most undesirable" carry the weight of stigma, but their use was informed by the dominant medical thinking of the time: hospital patients with already compromised immune systems needed to be protected from TB sufferers. Not surprisingly, Health Commissioner Stanley concurred on the need for such a facility. In May 1913, he expressed his concern that foreigners who did not have the means to go to a "proper sanatorium at home"—meaning in Europe—also lived in conditions where tuberculosis would continue to spread (SMA U1-16-617). Commissioner Stanley recommended a budget provision for the following year to allow a small hospital to be built on a corner of the Municipal Isolation Hospital grounds.

The need for a hospital was echoed by the secretary of the King's Daughters Society, an organization that provided aid to poor foreigners in Shanghai, including extra nutrition for about 50 tuberculosis cases who were residing at home. In May 1913, a letter from the society's secretary pointed out that many poor foreigners were at risk from the conditions in which they lived. Owing to high rents, these individuals were forced

> to live in small Chinese or semi-foreign houses in crowded alleyways or narrow streets, surrounded by Chinese amongst whom the disease is, as is well known, very widespread. They are for the most part very poor, underfed and underclothed, and have large families; as a rule, the whole family is housed in two or three rooms. These crowded insanitary conditions are exactly those which make for the development and spread of tuberculosis. ("Suggested Consumption Hospital" 1913: 228)

The King's Daughter's Society pointed out that these individuals posed a threat to wider society and implored the government to hospitalize advanced cases and build a sanatorium to isolate milder cases.

As the passage above illustrates, some of the language used to refer to Chinese citizens and their homes demonstrates colonial disdain toward the native population. Indeed, the SMC was much more concerned about the health of foreign residents than that of their Chinese neighbors. In the views of both the SMC health commissioner and the secretary of the King's Daughters Society, Shanghai was largely unhygienic, and the SMC had a moral obligation to intervene. As in other places around the world, TB tracked along socioeconomic lines. Individuals with more means had more access to space for rest and exercise, as well as lower incidence of the disease. Based on overall numbers, the poorest residents of Shanghai tended to be Chinese, so it is not surprising that deaths among Chinese were higher than those among foreigners; however, there was socioeconomic stratification in both the Chinese and the foreign populations. The status of poor foreigners in the International Settlement was somewhat contested since they were not ratepayers, but the health department felt obligated to help them.

Certainly, creating isolated TB facilities would benefit individuals without adequate financial means. Poor foreigners included Eurasians, Portuguese, and Sikhs, as well as White Russians and Jews who fled the pogroms. SMC correspondence advised that at least 50 free beds were needed. Moreover, should such a facility be created, "At first, the majority of cases will be of a more or less hopeless character, but later on, cases will come forward at an earlier stage with corresponding benefit to themselves and others" (SMA U1-16-617). Indeed, the health department recognized that TB had advanced to a point where many were gravely ill, particularly among the poor. The disease burden was large, so it was going to take time to bring high tuberculosis prevalence under control. Ironically, it was this point that led to the initial rejection of the sanatorium the first time it came up for a vote before the SMC ratepayers. Despite near-unanimous agreement among civil servants, representatives of charitable organizations, and doctors, the special resolution to build a hospital was voted down in March 1914, prompting redoubled efforts by the health department.

In preparation for a new vote in March 1915, the *North China Daily News* report highlighted the social determinants of health, much as international anti-TB associations did for their supporters. The report emphasized that the TB Question was closely tied to the cycle of poverty; it was "aggravated by the fact that poverty compels most of the patients to remain at their work as long as possible, thus greatly increasing the field of infection" ("Tuberculosis Hospital" 1915: 94). Ultimately, the disease had the potential to deepen poverty by compromising the ability to work. Thus, TB became framed as a moral hazard upon which the council would be forced to act, and it finally did. At the ratepayers' meeting in March 1915, the motion carried to build a new wing to the isolation hospital. But this does not mean that TB control suddenly became a priority.

As the SMC ratepayers were slow in approving the hospital wing, the SMC was slow in bringing those plans to fruition. Eventually, a foundation for a TB ward was prepared on the grounds of the Municipal Isolation Hospital, and the facility was scheduled to be completed in 1917, but it was small and did not open until 1919 (SMA U1-16-617). Even in 1919, discussion continued about renovation and staffing to allow for more patients to be served. For instance, at the annual ratepayers' meeting in 1919, Health Officer Arthur Stanley reported on the Municipal Isolation Hospital: "The old pavilion is in the course of alteration to provide for the reception of tuberculosis cases, and should be ready in June, or as soon as a nursing staff can be provided" ("Health Department" 1919:

Tuberculosis and the Quest for Modernity

123). Indeed, lack of a dormitory on site for nurses was one of the main factors delaying the opening of the facility. Following the end of the war in Europe, more staff were finally available to travel to Shanghai, and the TB hospital finally began receiving visitors in December 1919. The October 1920 *HOR* reported that "the foundation of satisfactory work against this greatest of world plagues may be said to have now been laid" (Stanley 1920b: 379).

During the wait for sanatorium approval, construction, and staffing, the SMC took a multipronged approach to TB prevention that resembled some of the tactics used by anti-TB associations elsewhere in the world. For instance, the October 1913 *Health Officer's Report* talks about use of lectures and handbills for Chinese residents explaining the way TB is spread (Stanley 1913b: 260). As was the case elsewhere globally, indiscriminate spitting was a point of contention. A Chinese-language handbill cautioned consumptives not to cough in others' faces and to avoid spitting. But the messages regarding spitting were mixed. Thus, even before the establishment of isolation facilities, there were attempts at social control of individual health behaviors. Health authorities cautioned individuals to avoid actions believed to dirty the streets, but whether spitting actually spread TB was a point of contention. In both 1913 and 1918, monthly *HORs* questioned the link between TB and spitting. In 1913, Health Officer Arthur Stanley wrote, "The spitting nuisance is relatively unimportant from the point of view of spreading consumption. The consumptive is the direct danger, and it is the fresh germs which are given out which sow the contagion. Once the spit is dried, the germs are mostly dead. It is obvious, therefore, that the main thing is to obtain fairly complete separation of infective consumptives" (1913a: 241). Likewise, in the January 1918 *Health Officer's Report*, Stanley argued:

> False ideas as to dirt cause attention to be distracted from more important matters. Dry dust is comparatively innocuous. The microbes of disease are mostly killed rapidly by drying. The danger of spitting in the street and its relation to the spread of Tuberculosis has been overdone. The bacillus of Tuberculosis when dried is soon killed, so that the probability of contracting the disease from dust blowing about in the street is remote. (1918a: 50)

In addition to preventive activities, government and other local actors sought to provide outpatient care to TB sufferers. The November 1913 *Health Officer's Report* outlines a plan for TB care using dispensaries. Indeed, it may seem odd that "dispensaries" should have played a role in the pre-antibiotic era; however, these facilities were not pharmacies. Instead, they functioned as grassroots clinics that allowed for interaction between medical personnel and the public, including Chinese citizens. Thus, they functioned much as dispensaries did elsewhere in the world (Bryder 1988; Teller 1988; Bates 1992). In Shanghai, every reported case received a visit from a nurse or health inspector who would note the housing conditions and whether TB sufferers were able to see a doctor. While dispensary employees did not make recommendations regarding living conditions, they did make treatment recommendations. If the patient was too poor to see a doctor, the SMC tuberculosis officer would visit them at home and advise on the most suitable treatment location, "whether at home, at the dispensary, the hospital or sanatorium" (Stanley 1913c: 292). For the final two recommendations, lack of beds was an ongoing problem.

Although the new hospital wing eventually provided an additional place to house foreign TB sufferers, it did not succeed in measurably reducing TB incidence among foreigners, or among Chinese residents. In fact, until 1928, the number of deaths from TB, particularly among the Chinese, was markedly higher than in 1911. By the late 1910s and early 1920s, it was not unusual for there to be more than 100 deaths from TB among the Chinese population of the International Settlement in a single week. Certainly, it is possible that cases and deaths from TB had actually remained relatively stable and statistical reporting simply became better as more attention was paid to TB. Regardless, on paper, the numbers certainly increased into the 1920s, and as the next section will highlight, governments began to pay a bit more attention.

Growing Commitment to Disease Control among Vulnerable Populations

By the early 1920s, there was finally growing government commitment to controlling TB. This commitment can be seen with respect to how TB was handled in two areas: the jail and factories employing children. TB control interventions helped in the jail, which can be seen as a microcosm of society. Many prisoners emanated from poor neighborhoods and were eventually released back into society, so they influenced societal disease prevalence and mortality more generally. This example illustrates how effective TB control interventions could be in a capacity with strict social control.

Infection rates were notably high among convicts (including both Chinese and foreigners). Both the SMC *Annual Report* for 1921 and a report published in 1922 highlighted the urgent need for interventions in the jail. This urgency arose from data emerging in the previous years. In October 1918 and November 1919, 159 convicts were examined, of whom 107 (or 67 percent) had evidence of lung disease (SMC 1922: 117A). Fully 18 percent of convicts were believed to suffer from active TB when they entered the jail. According to the December 1922 report, between 1918 and 1921, an astounding 72.29 percent of deaths in the jail were from TB, including 9 in 10 the previous year (1922: 448). The report noted that general conditions of sanitation, cleanliness, and ventilation were better than most convicts were accustomed to, so some other factor must be at work:

Tuberculosis and the Quest for Modernity 43

> The majority of these patients are underfed and put on weight very fast during the first months of imprisonment; and it seems likely that, if active cases could be detected early and treated for two or three months with rest and feeding, and thereafter given work in a special section of the Gaol under medical supervision, many more would survive their sentence. (SMC 1922: 118A)

The jail then implemented a series of regulations for the detection of TB, including quarantine observation cells to prevent the spread of infection. Other interventions were attempted, as well. Perhaps most important was a reconsideration of convicts' diets and the addition of more protein.

This situation was notable for two reasons. First, the jail was a total institution where the effect of interventions could be seen. The primary concern seems to be in making sure that jails were humane places, which were not akin to a death sentence from infectious disease. Additionally, many inmates would eventually be released, so concern about them was also concern about their communities. As the long quotation above illustrates, most of the convicts—certainly most of the convicts stricken with TB—were poor. Many were malnourished, which had likely increased their susceptibility to TB and impaired their bodies' ability to fight infection when it occurred. The improved nutrition they received would not continue after their release; malnourishment was likely a wider concern. Thus, releasing infectious former prisoners back into these communities threatened disease recurrence. This was one of the first times SMC health interventions specifically targeted a vulnerable population with respect to the social determinants of health.

Looking beyond the jails, some of the SMC's attention also started to shift toward factory conditions. As an example, the Child Labor Commission was formed in 1923 and surveyed the situation of child employment making observations and recommendations based on internationally accepted child labor norms. Among the survey's important findings, the minimal monthly cost of living for a household exceeded the wages that men and women in several professions (e.g., coolies and sorters) could make, necessitating the employment of additional household members, including children. Factories were particularly pernicious places for children, because of the humidity of workshops, which was believed to aggravate the spread of TB. Some children entered the factories not as employees but brought by mothers who did not have access to childcare. Consequently, "rows of baskets containing babies and children, sleeping or awake as the case may be, lie placed between the rapidly moving and noisy machinery" (Child Labor Commission 1924: 261). The children who did work often faced difficult conditions. For instance, they had to stand all day; in silk factories, they had to reach into basins of nearly boiling water to retrieve silkworm cocoons. The report admonished that neither the central government nor the

SMC had the power to enact labor regulations, but it made recommendations anyway, including setting the minimum age of employment at 14 in factories with dangerous machines, limiting shifts to 12 hours, and prohibiting overnight work for children (Child Labor Commission 1924: 268–69). While the work on child labor in Shanghai really did not mature until the late 1920s, it represented an area of growing concern (Jackson 2017).

By the time the Nanjing government assumed office, the amount of official attention devoted to health and TB had started to shift. In 1926, 150 inpatients and 9,972 outpatients received treatment in the tuberculosis block of Shanghai's Municipal Isolation Hospital, a facility with only 42 beds for TB patients (SMA U1-16-148; U1-16-654; U1-16-656).[9] Starting in 1927, the monthly *HOR*s also reported on a free outpatient tuberculosis clinic. The January 1927 *Public Health Report* estimated that there had been 11,000 cases among Shanghai's Chinese residents. Likewise, the report estimated that about 10 percent of all deaths were from tuberculosis, and 30 percent of deaths among working-age adults were from TB. While this clinic was expressly for examination, diagnosis, and observation of foreign cases, its efforts in two areas went beyond the foreign community: it provided education, and it sent personnel to examine the living arrangements of TB sufferers. Thus, staff began observing some of the more crowded spaces in the city, which were occupied by both Chinese and foreigners. Indeed, by 1927, commitment to tuberculosis control was growing; however, in April 1928, the health officer noted, "TB seems rather to have been shouldered out of sight by other more urgent health problems," but it "presents a problem which will eventually have to be faced" (Jordan 1928: 210).

Conclusion

In nations around the globe, controlling TB was part of the early twentieth-century Progressive movement. The notion of progress was often exported from more developed countries to less developed countries, including colonies. Westerners believed they were enlightened and, thus, had a responsibility to spread this knowledge widely, but their ideas met with resistance in the countries where they were being imposed. China was no exception. Its swift and decisive response to the 1910–1911 Manchurian plague outbreak demonstrated that it was capable of tackling its own medical emergencies. The Chinese government and various health organizations then conflicted and cooperated with international health organizations throughout the following decades. TB was much more widespread but was slower acting than diseases like plague, cholera, and

---

9. After the Municipal Council Sanatorium was founded, the isolation hospital reduced the number of designated TB beds to 24.

smallpox, so Shanghai's colonial government did not prioritize its control. While a TB wing eventually opened at the Municipal Isolation Hospital, social reformers recognized that TB's causes were deeply rooted in the inequalities that arose with modernization; thus, stopping TB was incompatible with economic development. This dilemma was not an easy one for China's reformers in the early twentieth century, just as it has not been easy for today's leaders.

2

An Unrealized Vision of Health and Tuberculosis Control, 1928–1949

On June 6, 1941, Chinese workers entered the Shanghai Anti-Tuberculosis Association's Shanghai Hospital and seized the operating table, stretchers, X-ray equipment, microscopes, and other furniture and equipment, such as beds. The commissioner of health of the Chinese administration, a representative of the local, collaborationist government, headed this operation to recover this loaned equipment, which was needed for another medical facility in Shanghai. During the seizure, SATA's hospital supervisor, Dr. Lee S. Huizenga, looked on helplessly (SMA U1-16-2660; U1-16-2664; and U38-1-191).[1] Following the incident, Huizenga promptly sent letters to the editors of local papers, urgently appealing to private citizens for help in replacing the lost equipment. A day later, local papers reported that this "tragedy" had turned into a "boon": locals flooded the organization with gifts of equipment and furniture, including the beds needed to ensure patients would not have to sleep on the floor (SMA U1-16-2660). Consequently, the hospital could continue its work, despite wartime equipment shortages.

This vignette illustrates several of the challenges in TB control during the twenty years leading up to the Communist victory in 1949. The two decades addressed in this chapter are often broken into three (or four) periods: the 1928–1937 "Nanjing Decade," the 1937–1945 war years, and the 1946–1949 postwar period. During the Nanjing Decade, the Guomindang government, which was based in Nanjing, wanted to implement a modern state, based on a Western model, with a genuine desire to unite and strengthen China. This state

---

1. Huizenga was a Dutch American medical missionary from Grand Rapids, MI, who served in China from 1920 until his death in a Japanese camp in Zhabei District in July 1945. After serving at the Shanghai Leprosarium, he became active with SATA at its founding. He served as superintendent of SATA's Tuberculosis Hospital, and as superintendent of hospitals after the superintendent of the Shanghai Hospital, Dr. Henry Chu, died in February 1941. Huizenga chaired SATA's publicity committee when it was founded in 1940 and served as general secretary of the organization.

emphasized development and modernization, but implementation of this vision varied based on resources and institutional capacity at locations throughout China. Growing conflict with the Japanese and public demonstrations against foreigners also punctuated the Nanjing Decade, including in Shanghai. As an example, in September 1931, the Japanese seized control of Manchuria without resistance, which prompted indignation and mass mobilization among students, merchants, and workers in Shanghai. Methods of resistance included demonstrations, marches, and boycotts, and some of the aggrieved parties even went to Nanjing to protest. In Shanghai, Japanese troops also attacked Zhabei for five weeks in late January to early March 1932, prompting mobilization in all sectors of society (Bergère 2009). The GMD government was divided on the approach to the Japanese, which complicated struggles over health-related resources. This chapter situates TB control with respect to various elements of the National Health Reconstruction program, which the Nanjing government sought to implement.

On paper, implementing a TB control plan dovetailed nicely with the GMD vision for health; however, there were many challenges with respect to implementation, including macro- and micro-level factors, as well as medical factors. At the macro level, its tenuous geopolitical hold on some areas compromised the GMD government's efforts to implement health interventions. Recent scholarship has demonstrated that some health interventions, such as vaccination, became widespread during the 1928–1937 Nanjing Decade in various Chinese locales and continued during the war (N. E. Barnes 2018; Nakajima 2018; Brazelton 2019b). In particular, cholera vaccination efforts continued in Shanghai and were a rare area of cooperation between Chinese and foreigners, including the Japanese occupiers. But the situation in occupied Shanghai was complex. As Nakajima (2018) writes, Chinese elites who wanted to improve the health of Chinese citizens had an ambiguous relationship with both Western colonialists and the Japanese. Many Chinese elites admired biomedicine and believed it could transform society. Likewise, the Japanese had largely adopted Western models of bacteriology and sought to implement health campaigns in areas of China. This raised ethical questions for local Chinese when it came to cooperating with Japanese health campaigns, such as cholera vaccination in 1938 (Nakajima 2018). Many in Shanghai accommodated the Japanese, perhaps because survival was their more immediate aim (Brook 2005).

Part of the chapter focuses on health interventions between August 1937 and August 1945. In China, the conflict taking place during this period is called the War of Resistance against the Japanese (抗日战争). In English, it is sometimes called the Second Sino-Japanese War to distinguish it from the First Sino-Japanese War, of 1894–1895. In this chapter, I refer to the period as the Japanese Occupation, because of the Japanese hold on Chinese parts of Shanghai (and parts of the International Settlement north of Suzhou Creek), starting with intense fighting between August and November 1937, known as the Battle of Shanghai. With the outbreak of war in 1937, the GMD government relocated from Nanjing to Chongqing. Many scholars further subdivide the war years in two: before the Japanese bombing of Pearl Harbor (1937–1941) and after the United States entered the war (1942–1945). Indeed, the struggle over resources in parts of Shanghai looked very different between 1938–1941 and 1942–1945. The early war years (1938–1941) are often called the "lonely island" (孤岛) period, a time of relative prosperity when some industry relocated from the Japanese-held areas in Zhabei, Hongkou, and Yangpu to the foreign concessions. By contrast, in the late war years (1942–1945), Japan also controlled the foreign concessions. After 1942, some Westerners, including Lee S. Huizenga, were held in camps, and others, such as SMC health commissioner J. H. Jordan, departed Shanghai. Archival records from 1942 to 1945 are not as complete as those from before 1941, but the records that do exist suggest that there was not a dramatic shift in implementation of TB control measures in 1942. As the opening vignette illustrates, the Japanese Occupation complicated but did not arrest the vibrant efforts in TB control that non-profit and private actors carried out, with some government support in 1937–1941. Moreover, as the chapter will illustrate, in 1942–1943 SATA proudly reported that all funding was being raised locally, when foreign funds were tied up supporting war efforts elsewhere around the globe.

The equipment seizure at SATA's Shanghai Hospital occurred five months prior to Pearl Harbor, and it illustrates several challenges in TB control before 1949. As highlighted in the previous chapter, before the discovery of effective antibiotics, isolation of sufferers was a commonly used disease control mechanism, including at the Shanghai Hospital, which had 60 beds, including 20 for paying patients, who helped to subsidize the costs of the less fortunate. Despite having been envisioned as a self-sufficient facility, during its 3.5-year affiliation with SATA, it always struggled for resources (Core 2019). In Shanghai, TB control involved cooperation between public and private entities, neither of whom had the resources or the mandate to fully implement TB control throughout a divided city. Certainly, this vignette illustrates the antagonistic relationship between collaborationist Chinese and a largely foreign-led organization. At first glance, it appears that the primary actors were SATA and the Chinese government, but SATA itself attempted to bring together multiple entities, not always successfully. SATA received support from both the Chinese national government as well as the local governments of Shanghai. Its funding came, in part, from grants-in-aid from both the French administration and the Shanghai Municipal Council, and it had a number of foreign doctors and donors among its leadership.

Additionally, the organization had close ties to other organizations involved in the tuberculosis movements internationally, as well as to business leaders, both locally and internationally. SATA actively sought to include Chinese nationals among its leadership and in its decision making, but as this example illustrates, Chinese loyalties were divided. At the time of the equipment seizure, the local Chinese government in Shanghai largely collaborated with the Japanese. During the equipment seizure, French police and the director of the Public Health Service of the French Municipal Council (FMC) were present because the hospital was in the French Concession. Perhaps the multiple actors could have united around the common cause of controlling the most widespread and deadly infectious disease, but resources, such as equipment and the space needed for disease control, were extremely limited. Consequently, conflict often ensued.

This chapter adds to the growing body of scholarship demonstrating that some health and welfare interventions, which would become hallmarks of the Mao era, originated under GMD rule (M. L. Bian 2005; Dillon 2015; N. E. Barnes 2018; Nakajima 2018; Tillman 2018; Brazelton 2019b; Soon 2020). Specifically, the chapter demonstrates that collection and use of disease statistics, hygiene campaigns, and expansion of health facilities and personnel for TB control originated before 1949. Health campaigns became relatively standard in Shanghai during the 1930s; however, my findings on TB prevention programming echo previous critiques that during the Nanjing Decade, TB control was pitched largely to the middle class, rather than those who needed it most (Lei 2010). Relatedly, TB control during this era did not pay enough attention to how interventions might be targeted to improve standards of living. While direct interventions were not made to raise the standard of living of the poor, benevolent actors did emphasize development of hospital and outpatient facilities to support poor TB patients. Nakajima (2018) and Tillman (2018) have both examined the expansion of nonprofits in Shanghai in the provision of health and welfare services before 1949. Likewise, N. E. Barnes (2018) has examined the expansion in the ranks of low-paid medical workers in developing medical services during the War of Resistance in free China. In occupied Shanghai, the state relied on private and voluntary organizations to provide many TB control services, both before and during the war.

Advances in science and technology prompted a dramatic shift in postwar disease control in 1946–1949. As the penultimate section of this chapter illustrates, during the postwar period, government, nonprofits, and other leaders cooperated to make medical advances more widely available. Specifically, the BCG vaccine, mass radiography, and effective antibiotics came into widespread usage as technologies that would revolutionize TB control. The postwar period was a prequel to systematic efforts to make medical advances widely available after 1949. Thus, this chapter echoes previous scholarship emphasizing continuity before and after 1949, as the state began to prioritize state medicine and build a national social welfare program (M. L. Bian 2005, Dillon 2015, Tillman 2018).

A National Vision for Health, 1928–1937

In 1928, the GMD was determined to unite and strengthen China by battling widespread disease. To this end, the GMD government developed a National Health Administration and worked closely with international organizations, such as the Rockefeller Foundation and League of Nations Health Organization, particularly in rural areas. The GMD also developed a national health reconstruction program, which had several elements upon which TB control efforts would build, including improved statistical monitoring, emphasis on preventive health, and modern scientific treatment. The GMD government also began to develop health infrastructure to implement its vision of health. This section provides an overview of each element of this vision.

National health reconstruction stressed monitoring of health statistics with creation of infrastructure to support this national program. During the 1930s and 1940s, the Chinese state made strides in compiling and monitoring statistics, including those associated with the human body. Scholars have argued that the collection of statistics was a crucial undertaking for creating citizenship and governing nations throughout the globe (Porter 1999; Foucault 2004; Lam 2011; DiMoia 2013). China's first concerted efforts to create and monitor health statistics based on infectious disease notification at the national level occurred during the Nanjing Decade. According to a 1928 Ministry of Health directive, doctors were required to report diagnoses of several prevalent infectious diseases to authorities within twelve hours, for example, typhoid, dysentery, cholera, smallpox, plague, diphtheria, meningitis, and scarlet fever (Yip 1995; Bu 2017). Thus, the program aimed to scale the sort of reporting that was done under the SMC Health Department to the national level. Despite its prevalence in the urban population, TB was not among the infectious diseases requiring notification in the initial 1928 directive; however, in Shanghai, a push was made to get a clearer picture of TB rates.

Likewise, national health reconstruction advocated for preventive health through environmental and personal hygiene. The GMD government was concerned about changing China's image as the "sick man of Asia" and viewed health education as one of the keys to making this a reality. In particular, in 1934, Chiang Kai-shek launched the New Life Movement, which encouraged individuals to become modern citizens by adopting hygienic habits and Confucian morality. This movement was premised on social control, as it encouraged transformation of health behaviors and state regulation of individual bodies. Several sites throughout the nation, including factories and schools, piloted health education programs aimed at changing individual health behaviors. While mass mobilization in health is considered a hallmark of Mao-era health campaigns, some aspects of health education programs, such as sending health professionals into schools and other workplaces to provide education, began in this era. Moreover, as other scholars have demonstrated, educational campaigns, such as lectures in urban venues, were fairly widespread. For instance, as Liping Bu illustrates, in the early 1930s, Beijing's hospital doctors delivered public lectures on topics including the benefits of public health and prevention of diseases such as trachoma, cholera, plague, and TB (Bu 2017). Likewise, in Shanghai, organizations carried out standardized campaigns, starting with opening ceremonies in large public venues (Nakajima 2018). Yet, as this chapter illustrates, one characteristic of TB educational materials of this era was that they sometimes aimed at donors who could invest in public health efforts, rather than the poor themselves.

National health reconstruction further emphasized "scientific medicine" (by which they meant Western biomedicine), expanding health infrastructure, and training medical personnel. Members of the Chinese intelligentsia, such as Kang Youwei, Liang Qichao, Chen Duxiu, and Lu Xun, wanted to promote scientific medicine.[2] Many Chinese officials also embraced Western biomedicine and began to develop infrastructure to support its adoption, including hospitals, outpatient clinics, laboratories, medical schools, and public health centers for providing preventive and curative services (Bowers 1974; Bu 2017). Efforts to staff this expanding infrastructure followed closely. The National Health Administration began to standardize requirements for physicians, dentists, pharmacists, nurses, and midwives and to train those personnel (Yip 1995; Andrews 2014; Grypma and Zhen 2014; N. E. Barnes 2018). Given the plurality of medical providers in China, estimating the number of health personnel was difficult. By any estimate, China had an acute need for trained medical professionals. According to one estimate, in the 1930s, China had one Western-style doctor for every 80,000 persons—compared to one doctor for every 1,500 persons in England and one doctor for every 800 persons in the United States (Hillier and Jewell 1983). Attempts were made to build and staff infrastructure in Shanghai, but as this chapter demonstrates, private and nonprofit actors, rather than the government, undertook much of this work with respect to TB.

Shanghai was supposed to be a national centerpiece, and it started to develop a health administration even before the National Health Administration was in

---

2. Lu Xun had a very personal connection to TB: his father died from TB, as he did in 1936. Lu, who had studied medicine in Japan and felt such traditional beliefs reflected badly on China, critiqued superstitious practices in his 1922 short story, "Medicine," (*Yao* 药). In the story, a couple purchase a steamed bun (*mantou*) dipped in the blood of a revolutionary martyr for their son who is dying from TB. At the time, this "medicine" was believed to be the elixir needed to cure TB, but in Lu Xun's story, the son dies anyway ([1922] 1972).

place. Efforts to develop a municipal health bureau (卫生局)[3] dovetailed nicely with the Greater Shanghai Plan, which sought to create a municipality to rival the concessions, starting in 1927 (MacPherson 1990; Jackson 2017). Chinese officials were eager to put their hygienic modernity on display by developing a health bureau modeled after the SMC Health Department and headed by foreign-trained Chinese, with impressive credentials and experience working with foreigners. The first director, Hu Hongji (胡鸿基), was a medical doctor who received a Rockefeller Foundation International Health Board Fellowship, which funded his training at the Johns Hopkins School of Public Health. After he returned to China, Hu served as the chief of vital statistics at a health station in Beijing (under John Grant), which informed his approach to community health (Jackson 2017, Nakajima 2018). Hu headed the bureau from 1927 until he died in a traffic accident in 1932. After Hu, Li Ting'an (李廷安) directed the bureau. Like Hu, Li held both a medical degree (from PUMC) and a doctorate in public health (from Harvard) and had worked in a health station (in Shanghai) (Nakajima 2018).

In Shanghai, the Chinese Health Bureau created an ambitious infrastructure development plan to provide care to all residents of the city—including a large general hospital and branch hospitals—but it was never realized because of lack of funding. One area where the bureau made some progress was in the development of community health stations. Health stations collected statistics, promoted health education, administered vaccines, monitored environmental sanitation, and offered free or inexpensive care at attached clinics; however, only 4 out of the 17 planned stations were built before 1937 (Nakajima 2018: 96). Like the SMC Health Department, the Chinese Health Bureau was grossly underfunded and had uneven success. It faced challenges dealing with some of the most basic health issues: two-thirds of its budget went to street sweeping and night soil removal (Nakajima 2018: 90). Likewise, the health bureau continued to struggle with the health effects of poverty, including a rise in unburied corpses. As Li Ting'an noted, in 1934 and 1935, his department picked up more than 100,000 coffins (T. Li 1935, Nakajima 2018).[4] Owing to the failure to address poverty, which is a root cause of tuberculosis, both government and nonprofit actors had only limited success in controlling the leading infectious disease.

---

3. In this chapter, I refer to the health bureau founded by the Chinese administration as the "Chinese Health Bureau," to distinguish it from the health departments of the foreign concessions. After 1949, only the Chinese health bureau remained , so I drop the "Chinese" distinction. In subsequent chapters, it is called "Shanghai Health Bureau," "municipal health bureau," or simply "health bureau."

4. Likewise, the number of exposed corpses collected in the International Settlement saw 3.5-fold increase between 1930 and 1937—from 5,796 to 20,796 (Jackson 2017: 200).

The Leading Infectious Disease

Under this backdrop of increased attention to health, two organizations specifically dedicated to TB control were founded in Shanghai: the National Anti-Tuberculosis Association of China (NATAC, 中国防痨协会) in 1933, and the Shanghai Anti-Tuberculosis Association (上海防痨协会) in 1938. Both organizations aimed to implement elements of national health reconstruction by focusing on the leading infectious disease of the era. NATAC and SATA were not the only health-related nonprofits active in Shanghai during the 1930s and 1940s, but they were resilient anti-disease organizations throughout the period, which survived to the present day. SATA was one of the only organizations to prioritize increasing beds in single-disease, TB-care facilities between the organization's 1938 founding and its Hospital Building and Equipment Fund Campaign, which ended in February 1942.

Understanding the scope of TB infections and death was one of the first steps in its control, but this was difficult to accomplish. When he announced the founding of the NATAC at the first Tuberculosis Conference of the China Medical Association in 1933, Shanghai's mayor, Wu Tiecheng (Wu Te-chen 吴铁城), estimated that China had an average of 1.2 million deaths annually from TB (T. Li 1934). As more attention became focused on TB after the formation of NATAC, it became clear that early estimates of annual deaths from TB were low. In NATAC's first annual report for 1934, Mayor Wu revised the estimate of annual deaths in China upward to 1.6 million (SMA U1-16-2659). Regardless, as Sean Lei has argued, "Precision of the numbers did not matter. . . . [They] were just tools for awakening the government and the Chinese people to this crisis of a national scale" (2010: 258). Likewise, enlisting the help of prominent political figures, at least symbolically, was a strategy used by organizations in various locations worldwide to raise the profile of anti-TB work (Knopf 1922).[5] The strategy also served to make policy makers aware of anti-TB work in the location they governed.

As the New Life Movement was launched and NATAC began its work, almost all adults in Shanghai had been exposed to TB. Results of a 1934 test to measure the endemicity of TB in Shanghai indicated a 60 percent infection rate for all age groups and a 94 percent exposure rate for all persons over the age of 24 (Andrews 1997). Certainly, not all exposed or infected persons developed active disease, but depending on their socioeconomic situation, many did. With limited treatment options, both in terms of medicine and isolation facilities, mortality was also high. According to the public health report of the concessions, in 1929,

---

5. For example, this strategy was used in the United States, where Grover Cleveland, Theodore Roosevelt, and Warren Harding all served as vice presidents of the NTA.

966 of 980,000 Chinese residents died from TB, or about 98.6 per 100,000. This report also stated that 41 percent of deaths from infectious disease were from TB (CMA 1997).

According to the most comprehensive data available, Shanghai saw improvements to TB indicators in the late 1920s and early 1930s. TB mortality among Chinese residents within Shanghai's foreign concessions improved 54 percent between 1926 and 1936—from 140.4 per 100,000 to 64.4 per 100,000 (H. Li 2014). These improvements paralleled improvements occurring elsewhere in the world, which began around the turn of the twentieth century. Scholars have debated whether pre-antibiotic improvements in TB mortality elsewhere in the world occurred as a result of improved standards of living and better nutrition, or public health interventions, such as isolating sick persons (McKeown 1976; Szreter 1988). This debate is also relevant to Shanghai; however, it is no easier to determine whether the primary factor driving decreased TB mortality in Shanghai was improved standard of living or public health interventions. During the period, Shanghai was better able to isolate some TB sufferers than to improve living standards for everyone. Thus, the gains against TB were uneven and were not always sustained.

In 1937–1945, war drove increased incidence and mortality.[6] During the Japanese Occupation, Shanghai's urban crowding became more acute. The Japanese bombing commenced on August 13, 1937. For the next several months, several hundred thousand mostly Chinese people became refugees when these bombs threatened or destroyed the industrialized parts of Shanghai, such as Zhabei and Yangshupu (Henriot 2006; Bergère 2009; Jackson 2017; Tillman 2018).[7] The number of refugees fleeing into the foreign concessions was estimated to be at least 250,000 in the fall of 1937, but the peak of the crisis did not come until the following year. During the single month of April 1938, "more than 150,000 refugees sought shelter" (Jackson 2017: 200). Many of these refugees were forced to live in crowded, unsanitary conditions, including 280 refugee camps in the foreign concessions, which made them susceptible to infectious disease (SMA U38-1-191 and U38-5-1625; Henriot 2006; Ristaino 2008; and Tillman 2018).[8]

Interestingly, after the refugee problem became less acute around 1939, deaths from TB continued to rise, though not as dramatically as in 1937–1938.

---

6. Increased TB mortality during wartimes has been a worldwide phenomenon, and has been reported in countries including The Netherlands and Great Britain (Dubos and Dubos [1952] 1987).

7. Yangshupu is in today's Yangpu District.

8. *SATA First Annual Report* (August 1939) and *Report of the Tuberculosis Hospital of The Shanghai Anti-Tuberculosis Association* (in SMA U38-1-191); *First Annual Report of the Shanghai Hospital of the SATA: January 1, 1939–December 31, 1939* (SMA U38-5-1625).

An Unrealized Vision of Health and Tuberculosis Control 55

Table 2.1: Deaths from communicable diseases in Shanghai's foreign concessions, 1937–1941

	Deaths from 7 diseases*	Deaths from TB	TB deaths as % of total	Increase in TB deaths over previous year
1937	1,895	1,161	37.99%	
1938	5,313‡	2,074	28.08%	78.64%
1939	2,819	2,759	49.46%	33.03%
1940	2,627	3,713	58.56%	34.58%
1941	3,548	4,503	55.93%	21.28%

* smallpox, cholera, typhoid, diphtheria, scarlet fever, flu, cerebrospinal fever.
‡ The 1938 figure is abnormally high due to 2,110 deaths from cholera and 1,947 from typhoid.
Source: SMA U1-16-2664.

As indicated in Table 2.1, number of deaths from TB among the resident population for 1938 increased 78.64 percent from 1937. Increases were only 33.03 percent in 1939, 34.58 percent in 1940, and 21.28 percent in 1941. According to a 1942 report, deaths from TB exceeded the combined total from seven other leading diseases in the International Settlement and French Concession in 1940 and 1941 (Table 2.1, SMA U1-16-2664). There were no reported data from the Chinese City during most of this time because the Chinese Health Bureau ceased operations for 40 months from November 1937 until March 1941 (Nakajima 2018: 112). However, the vast majority of residents in all three sectors of the city were Chinese, so data from the Chinese City would likely similarly reflect rising mortality. On September 17, 1942, a *Shanghai Times* article predicted that the number of deaths from TB in the municipality would be even higher in 1942. The article drew upon an interview with SATA's general secretary, Dr. Lee S. Huizenga, who estimated a 70 percent infection rate. Only about 6 percent of residents throughout the municipality were believed to suffer from active disease, but this is still an astounding figure (SMA U1-16-2660).[9]

In addition to war, a potential factor driving increased incidence was that organizations specifically dedicated to TB control paid more focused attention and had a greater ability to identify cases, allowing more infections and deaths to make their way into statistical reporting. In the 1920s, case notification had been poor at best, and this contributed to inaccurate mortality numbers. The cause of

---

9. September 7, 1942, *Shanghai Times* article "Tuberculosis Said Rising in Shanghai; Prevalence of Disease Given Analysis." in SMA U1-16-2660.

death was known and reported only when sick persons made their way into the formal health system and were diagnosed. That cause of death was unknown in the majority of cases implies either that the deceased had not sought medical advice, or that medical personnel had failed to make a diagnosis. Either of these scenarios is likely. Reasons for failing to seek medical attention may have included fear of costs associated with the illness, including loss of livelihood, or fear of being diagnosed with a deadly disease when there was little hope for a cure. Isolating TB sufferers also entailed inconveniencing one's family, by isolating in the home or leaving for a sanatorium. For persons with no prior experience in the health system, general fear of the unknown might have also prevented them from seeking medical advice. Given that hospital resources, including personnel, had extremely limited capacity to receive patients and make standardized diagnoses the Shanghai Municipal Council Health Department concluded, "It is absurd to suppose that the figures of 'cases notified' include more than a fraction of the cases actually occurring" (SMA U1-16-714).

More resources being focused on TB control led to better diagnosis and case notification, specifically within the International Settlement and French Concession. Consequently, the number of cases notified as a percentage of total estimated cases improved in the 1930s. SATA publications listing statistical data also comment on this phenomenon. The *SATA Bulletin* for October through December 1942 states, "Someone jokingly said that it was the Shanghai Anti-Tuberculosis Association that boosted up the statistics" (SMA U38-1-191). Collecting data on disease cases is difficult even in times of peace, so it is unsurprising that the program probably never provided a full and accurate picture of the TB caseload. Regardless, the data began to illuminate the gravity of TB infection rates, which led to calls for action. Unlike the SMC, which Chapter 1 illustrated was primarily concerned about the economy, the Guomindang government devoted some attention to the poor, but disease control interventions did not always make it to the strata of the population where it was most needed.

Class-Biased TB Prevention

A second element of national health reconstruction was an emphasis on prevention. During a disease outbreak, widespread education emphasizing how individual behavior bears on the collective might help to change health behaviors, with the goal of limiting the spread of the disease. As an example, in the recent COVID-19 outbreak, individuals were invited to consider how their decisions regarding social distancing, mask wearing, or vaccination contribute to overall infection rates in their community. In the early 1930s health campaigns aimed at cleanliness became a vibrant part of Shanghai's TB control. These campaigns largely subscribed to the formulaic approach involving a public opening ceremony and widespread dissemination of written materials. However, this section investigates the mismatch between who was targeted in the health education campaigns and who was most susceptible to TB.

During the Nanjing Decade, indiscriminate spitting became an early target of TB control campaigns.[10] An anti-spitting week, conducted from March 28 to 31, 1934, was among NATAC's first efforts at implementing a mass prevention model. An opening ceremony at the Metropol Theatre launched the campaign. The campaign also involved Boy Scouts distributing handbills at intersections of major streets and days when educational programming targeted students, merchants, and factory workers (SMA U1-16-2659). Similar campaigns were held in 1935 and 1936. In addition to the anti-spitting campaigns, health professionals gave talks, both on the radio and in public settings. In 1934, six doctors spoke on the gospel radio station, one every two weeks for three months. Fifty public lectures, with an estimated total attendance of 7,500, were also given on Saturday nights and in colleges and schools (SMA U1-16-2659; Core 2014).

Unfortunately, several elements of these early prevention campaigns would have reached only the middle class. For example, both the space and time of the opening ceremony limited involvement. Although the event was free, a theater might not have felt welcoming to poor citizens. Holding the opening ceremony at 10:00 a.m. on a weekday would have also precluded involvement by waged workers, unless they worked the evening shifts. Lectures in schools and factories aimed to reach a wider audience but still missed large swaths of the population, such as families who did not have a member affiliated with the school and workers without stable factory employment. Certainly, radio campaigns aimed to reach a wider audience than public lectures did, but their effectiveness depended on access to electricity, radios, and broadcasts in dialects and language understandable to laypersons (Core 2014). In short, NATAC campaigns were largely ineffective in reaching those who did not participate in the formal-sector economy, including the urban poor.

As part of the anti-spitting weeks, as well as other times, NATAC created written materials, such as fliers, but the effectiveness of these materials is also questionable. Without illustrations specifically geared for a semiliterate public, written materials were probably only partially understood. For instance, one flier from the period depicts a snake, mostly hidden in grass. The flier has a cryptic title, "Hidden Disaster," designed to pique the curiosity of a literate public (NATAC n.d.). It educates its reader about the symptoms of TB—tired spirit,

---

10. While today modern epidemiologists recognize that TB is actually transmitted through *Mycobacterial tuberculosis* present in droplets when persons with active TB cough, at this time (and well into the 1950s), indiscriminate spitting in public places was thought to be a primary culprit because dried spittle could be kicked up and inhaled.

loss of weight and appetite, coughing, chest pain, and blood in one's saliva—to drive home the point that only doctors can uncover the hidden danger. While this message becomes clear as one reads the flier's text, it likely would not have reached workers who had not had the opportunity to attend school; literacy rates among the working class were not high in Shanghai during this time. In 1950, an estimated 34.5 percent of workers had attended elementary school, and 46 percent were believed to be illiterate (Gardner 1969). Literacy rates among the urban poor, such as peasant migrants, were likely even lower. Thus, the presence of so many written materials suggests a mismatch with the needs of the population. Despite living in conditions that made them susceptible to TB, workers and the urban poor were not the intended audience of the prolific written materials. It was not until population of focus shifted and workers became more privileged in the 1950s that preventive education would have a lasting effect.

Indeed, the education campaigns were out of step with the growing population of Shanghai. In the 1920s and 1930s, the city expanded rapidly as peasants escaped the poverty of the countryside. Many of these migrants eked out an existence through informal means and manual labor. The poor included an estimated 20,000 beggars, 50,000–60,000 dock workers, and more than a 100,000 rickshaw pullers (H. Lu 1999). An estimated fewer than 10 percent of Shanghai's citizens were lucky enough to find stable factory employment, and those who did faced deplorable conditions. In 1929, the city had 2,326 factories employing more than 285,000 workers, more than a third of them in the cotton spinning industry (Honig 1986). In textile factories, machinery whirred 24 hours a day, six days a week. Workers staffed looms in 12-hour shifts, alternating weekly between day and evening shifts for the duration of their two-year contract. Long hours and poor ventilation in the mills put workers at risk for respiratory diseases, and workers hesitated to take time off for illness because they would have to add two days to one month to the end of their contract for every sick day they missed. Consequently, minor health problems often advanced to more serious conditions. Those from outside Shanghai often lived in crowded dormitories, which may have exacerbated disease outbreaks. Locals who worked in the mills put their families at risk because many of them lived and slept in one room with numerous family members.

Because of the Japanese invasion, NATAC largely curtailed prevention efforts and outreach between August 1937 and October 1939, but SATA picked up the mantle (SMA U1-16-2659).[11] Like NATAC, SATA held an anti-TB week or similar activity on an annual basis. SATA cooperated with the Joint Committee

---

11. When the NATAC *Quarterly Journal* began to be printed, again, in October 1939, it noted: "The time is opportune for revival of activities on a modest scale." The organization clarified that "modest scale" meant that it would leave establishment of hospitals and sanatoria to its local branches.

of the Shanghai Women's Organizations on its March 1939 anti-spitting campaign, which involved radio talks, school visits by campaign staff, and dissemination of posters and buttons (SMA: U1-16-2659, U1-16-2664, and U38-1-191). In part, because of these efforts, the SMC codified several new health bylaws, including one governing spitting in June 1941: "No person shall spit in public places, public vehicles, streets or pavements, or in any other place where spitting is detrimental to public health" (SMA U38-5-1091).[12] But the law applied only to the International Settlement, and the meager CN$5 fine did not prove to be much of a deterrent. A retired health provider told me that when fines were first enacted, some violators chose to pay double, so they could spit again later (Provider 32). This humorous anecdote illustrates the futility of trying to change ingrained health behaviors.

SATA tried to bring about better compliance to the new law by coordinating with governments, schools, and various businesses in the community in an October 1941 campaign. Preparation for the campaign included contacting Chinese, English, and French daily newspapers about publicity; arranging Chinese and English radio broadcasts and talks in schools; producing and distributing Chinese posters to schools, buses, trams, and shops; and printing 30,000 Chinese and 12,000 English appeal letters. The Campaign Publicity Committee also had a photographer visit SATA's hospitals so pictures could be included in campaign publications (SMA U1-16-2664). At a meeting on September 1, 1941, publicity committee members reported that 28 Chinese radio stations would each reserve two to five spots daily for free. In the weeks immediately prior to the campaign, SATA representatives sought approval from SMC officials for bilingual banner slogans, which were printed on cloth donated from Wing On textiles (SMA U1-16-2665). This campaign also included lectures at 10 schools—5 in the International Settlement and 5 in the French Concession—including primary and secondary schools, as well as universities. Printed lectures were sent to other schools (SMA U1-16-2664).

While some of this publicity undoubtedly reached poorer residents, in several ways the intended audience for this campaign was still largely the literate public. In fact, while some of SATA's members approached the poor from a benevolent perspective, others lacked sensitivity to systemic inequality. As an example, at a meeting of SATA's publicity committee in preparation for a campaign, one member condescendingly mentioned targeting "the congested quarters" in a manner appropriate for reaching "ignorant people unable either to read or write" (SMA U1-16-2664). The example suggests that some victim blaming occurred, but the committee also strategized about how to begin to

---

12. National Anti-Tuberculosis Association of China (July) 1941, "Anti-Spitting Bylaw," *Quarterly Bulletin* 4(3): 8 (in SMA U38-5-1091).

reach the poor. This committee believed the help of students, YMCA secretaries, and church auxiliaries should be enlisted. A few efforts were made to target the most vulnerable groups, such as health talks, lectures, and demonstrations given in the refugee camp at Jiaotong University, but more outreach was needed (Sze 1937–1938).

SATA used two other types of written materials to attempt to raise awareness for the cause. One was also employed elsewhere in the world: Christmas / New Year seal contests campaigns. The 1938 Christmas Seal campaign was one of SATA's first activities after its founding: 7,000 sheets of 50 seals were printed, and the first campaign raised more than CN$4,500 in local currency (SMA U38-1-191).[13] Charity seals had previously been used in China, but these were the first anti-TB seals. As Margaret Tillman notes, Christmas tended to be a time that (foreign and Christian) benefactors in Shanghai opened their pockets. After the war, SATA switched to issuing seals at the Lunar New Year rather than Christmas because the organization deemed it more culturally appropriate in the Chinese context.

SATA also held a bilingual essay contest for high school and college students. High school and college students wrote essays on the topic "What Can the High School (or College) Student do in TB Control." SATA's first essay contest was held in 1941 and received a total of 22 Chinese essays and 21 English essays from students in three colleges and 10 high schools; eight monetary prizes were awarded: first and second prizes in Chinese and in English were granted for both high school and college students (SMA U1-16-2661). This contest helped to generate interest among a small portion of the populace; it was designed to get students to think about how they could contribute to TB control. The ideas generated through these essays could then be incorporated in future prevention activities. Such a contest was successful in that it facilitated retention of health information among participants, but obviously only literate persons could participate.

Of other written materials, some were aimed at potential donors to the organization rather than persons most at risk for disease. Pitching to the wealthy was a strategy employed to bring in funds. NATAC (and later SATA) hoped to activate the "humanitarian ideal of helping the sick and needy" (Nakajima 2018: 73). In 1935–1936, NATAC published a bilingual *Quarterly Bulletin* with news on TB control in cities nationwide, including Ningbo, Shaoxing, Suzhou, and Kunming (SMA U1-16-2659, U1-16-2662, and U38-5-1091).[14] SATA created a similar bulletin in 1942 and other written materials for educated citizens. Some

---

13. "Report of the Appeals Committee" in SATA's 1939 *First Annual Report*.
14. This bulletin had a circulation of 1,500 when it started to be published in 1934. Circulation expanded to 5,000 in 1935 and 8,000 in 1936. Publication stopped for two years during the Japanese occupation, and began again in 1939.

An Unrealized Vision of Health and Tuberculosis Control 61

of the earliest pamphlets and brochures included a three-by-six-inch, five-page booklet called *The Birth of the SATA*. Published during SATA's first fiscal year, the booklet appeals to emotion. It describes the thousands of war refugees "with their meager belongings" who flooded into the city, the "sick, carried upon doors." The sick and well were "compelled to sleep on the streets of the city until slowly spaces could be found to shelter them from the cold" (SMA U38-1-191[2]). This particular pamphlet had the goal of raising funds rather than awareness of disease symptoms.

The examples of NATAC and SATA illustrate that these nonprofit organizations implemented preventive programming in line with national health reconstruction, but this section has demonstrated that programming tended to be understood by the middle class and potential donors, rather than those most susceptible to TB. Some efforts were made to reach those in "congested quarters," who were sometimes viewed with colonial disdain. By 1942, resources for education became strained. For instance, the reports of the general secretary and Publicity Committee for April 1942–February 1943, note that publicity had been done "only on a limited scale," owing to the high cost of paper and printing (SMA U1-16-2661: 140). At the time, many foreign nationals were departing Shanghai, but continuing to operate treatment facilities remained a goal. As the next section details, local governments and private individuals built facilities for isolating TB sufferers and continued to staff them, even during the war.

Expanding Treatment during the Japanese Occupation, 1937–1945

A third element of national health reconstruction was the expansion of medical facilities and the promotion of scientific medicine. Since antibiotics effective in controlling TB were not discovered until 1943, increasing the number of isolation beds and outpatient treatment centers was central to TB control in Shanghai, across China, and throughout the world. In the late 1920s and early 1930s, facilities to isolate both Chinese and foreign TB sufferers were founded. Larger specialized facilities for TB patients tended to be built away from the city center because the disease was infectious (Provider 17).

As the Nanjing Decade began, Shanghai's government and private leaders recognized the acute need for beds. As detailed in Chapter 1, the SMC finally opened a TB isolation ward on the grounds of the Municipal Isolation Hospital in December 1919; however, immediately before formation of the Nanjing Government, the situation remained dire. On October 13, 1927, the assistant commissioner of public health of the SMC declared:

> The present system of treating Pulmonary Tuberculosis in Shanghai is a disgrace to medical science. The TB Block of the Isolation Hospital is merely a

dumping ground for dying persons or a transitory home for Consumptives before they can be moved elsewhere. . . . With regard to measures against the terrible scourge of TB, the Shanghai area is thirty years behind any other city of equivalent importance. (SMA U1-16-148)

Given this known deficiency, another facility for foreigners was planned in November 1927 and approved in June 1928 with 30 beds, which would increase in future years. In 1930, the facility had 36 beds: 2 for first-class, 2 for second-class, and 32 for free cases (SMA U1-16-655). The facility also later included 12 beds for children (SMA U1-16-617). Despite the fact that this Municipal Council Sanatorium admitted only foreign residents of the International Settlement (and a few from the French Concession), the facility was almost always full (SMA U1-16-654). In SMC correspondence, the hospital superintendent highlighted the strong demand: "I have a long waiting list" (SMA U1-16-654: 68). Relatives of both foreign and Chinese TB sufferers sent pleas to the commissioner of health requesting that beds be made available (SMA U1-16-617, SMA U1-16-655, and SMA U1-16-656).[15] Excessive demand eventually caused the SMC to limit length of stay, but this would not happen until 1935.

When NATAC first began its work, it focused on providing some outpatient services to compensate for the dearth of beds. NATAC opened its first TB clinic on June 1, 1934. The facility was open two hours each afternoon, six days a week, to provide free outpatient medical care. Within its first seven months of operation, it received 634 visits (SMA U1-16-2659). This low number—fewer than 100 visits per month, or only four to five cases per weekday—suggests that NATAC reached only a sliver of estimated cases in the city. More facilities and wider publication of available services were needed. In 1935, NATAC opened an additional clinic and gained permission to open more in Shanghai Municipal Council's branch health offices. In the summer of 1937, NATAC was raising funds so it could open the Yu Ya Ching TB Sanitarium with 150 beds and more clinics. Unfortunately, widespread bombing by the Japanese starting in August curtailed these efforts.

Private citizens also made efforts to establish hospitals with designated TB treatment beds, founding three facilities in today's Jing'an District, including a 24-bed hospital on Daxi Road in 1933, the Dongwu Hospital on Wanhangdu Road, and the pulmonary sanatorium on West Nanjing Road (Yin 2000). Larger facilities included the Chengzhong Hospital, which was founded in Yangpu District in 1933, and the Hongqiao (Hungjao 虹桥) Sanatorium, founded in

---

15. Municipal correspondence includes discussion of a plea from the relative of a prominent official in the Chinese Nationalist government for treatment in one of the first-class beds in June 1930. Because of her Chinese nationality, she was told to seek treatment in the Shanghai Tuberculosis Sanatorium on today's Yanan Road.

1934 (CMA 1997). Ding Huikang, son of the well-known proponent of Western medicine, Ding Fubao, founded the Hongqiao Sanatorium.[16] TB was a priority for the Ding family, owing to family history with the disease. Ding Fubao had TB but recovered; however, his father and one of his sons died from the disease (Andrews 2014). Consequently, Ding Huikang devoted himself to tuberculosis, founding both the Shanghai Tuberculosis Sanatorium and later the Hongqiao Sanatorium. When the Hongqiao Sanatorium was built, the main structure was a four-story building with southern-facing wards and private sun porches so patients could get fresh air.

War impacted several TB isolation facilities. In September 1937, Japanese planes power-dove over the Hongqiao Gardens, where the SMC Sanatorium was located. Machine gun nests believed to be located in the garden were the direct target; however, on the early morning of September 5, planes flew low enough for the sanatorium's night watch to see the pilots. The north side of the hospital block sustained a direct shell hit, and large sections of the ceiling plaster fell, forcing the facility to close (SMA U1-16-654).[17] Likewise, the Chengzhong Hospital also sustained damage during the air raids and closed, while the Hongqiao Sanatorium moved and continued to function (SMA U1-16-654; CMA 1997; Qiao 2020).[18] Relocation caused the Hongqiao Sanatorium to downsize. Before the war it had 100 beds, and in 1939, it had 75 beds, including 15 first-class, 28 second-class, 22 third-class, and 10 free beds (SMA U1-16-2661). During the war, Shanghai's need for TB treatment became even more acute when the Japanese bombing left hundreds of thousands of Chinese homeless.

After its founding, SATA surveyed the number of hospital beds in Shanghai designated for TB patients and presented results at the second Medical Committee meeting on January 26, 1939. According to this committee's findings, Shanghai had 19 facilities, with 529 beds designated for TB patients: 90 first-class, 167 second-class, 217 third-class, and 55 free beds (SMA U1-16-2661). SATA's survey was intended to be a starting place for study and action, so it was neither scientific nor comprehensive. Notably, in the table of results, the numbers of beds of each type in the various facilities do not add up to the totals listed at the bottom of the page. A handwritten addition of the "Great Shanghai Sanitarium" was also made at the end of the typed survey, which leads the critical viewer to wonder which

---

16. Ding Fubao translated at least 83 medical volumes from Japanese, widely published journal articles, and established a publishing company in Shanghai (Andrews 2015).

17. The closure of this Sanatorium did not reduce available beds for too long. In 1941 correspondence, the SMC's Superintendent of Hospitals claimed that there were nearly as many TB beds as before the war. Instead of 36 beds at the Sanatorium and 22 beds at the Municipal Isolation Hospital, in 1941, the SMC supported 33 beds in a general hospital and 25 in a facility on Brenan Road (SMA U1-16-617).

18. The Hongqiao Sanatorium's new location is now part of the Xuhui District Central Hospital.

other facilities might have been missed. To my knowledge, the survey missed at least one: the Russian Orthodox Confraternity's Hospital had a TB ward with 16 beds and continued to function during the early war years (SMA U1-16-617).[19]

Despite statistical imperfections, the data on hospitalization facilities suggest that beds disproportionately favored paying patients. Notably, not a single facility with free beds was exclusively free. Four of the five facilities with free beds—Grouchy, Hongqiao, Nanyang, and Paulun—had considerably more beds for paying than for free patients. Thus, there was only limited capacity for supporting those most vulnerable. The survey also investigated whether pneumothorax, X-rays, and specialists were available at each of the facilities. Pneumothorax, a surgical procedure which collapsed the lung in an attempt to immobilize it and allow for healing, was intended to facilitate shorter hospital stays, which could make beds available for others who needed them (SMA U1-16-617). Another takeaway from the survey was that specialists' skills could be used for outpatients, thus extending the reach of medical professionals beyond the few who were lucky enough to secure hospital beds. Based on the data, SATA worked to increase beds, personnel, and technology to try to reach more poor patients.

The distribution of beds in Shanghai, which prioritized treatment for paying patients, resembled that elsewhere in China. A survey of 30,000 TB patients at the Canton Hospital (in 1914–1925, 1929–1931) and David Gregg Hospital for Women (in 1927–1930) found that the

> tuberculosis infection rate was actually three times higher among patients in private rooms than among patients in wards. Since a stay in the wards cost about one-tenth to one-half of a stay in a private room, these data suggested that tuberculosis was much more prevalent among upper class patients than among the poor. This surprising discovery was confirmed by an analysis based on occupational groups: infection rates among professionals were more than three times higher than those among laborers. Rather than being determined by wealth, susceptibility to tuberculosis seemed to be connected to how a person spent his or her days. (Lei 2010: 260)

If data from the survey are accurate, the findings of higher TB infection rates among China's upper classes varied from those in other global locations. For instance, David Barnes (1995) found that in late-nineteenth and early twentieth-century France, domestic workers and those who patronized the cabaret had high TB prevalence and became targets of the anti-TB movement. Likewise, William Johnston highlights that in the 1920s, Japan's Anti-TB League paid attention to the more distal factors contributing to widespread TB: poor nutrition and long

---

19. The superintendent of this hospital wrote to Dr. W.R. Johnston, superintendent of SMC hospitals on April 16, 1938, to introduce his hospital's work, including the advantages of pneumothorax, and to propose solutions to the problem of TB treatment.

An Unrealized Vision of Health and Tuberculosis Control 65

working hours. If China's upper classes were really most susceptible to TB, the country is an outlier. An alternative explanation for the high prevalence of TB patients in private rooms would be that when demand for the few available beds was great, patients from upper-middle-class families had the knowledge and connections to advocate for themselves and procure a spot. Hospital administrations may have also relied on paying patients in the first- and second-class rooms to subsidize patients in the wards that offered beds on a charitable or semi-charitable basis. Certainly, SATA employed this strategy at its Shanghai Hospital.

While TB prevention efforts remained largely relegated to the middle class and potential donors, SATA prioritized treatment of poor TB patients as part of its mission. On January 18, 1938, professionals who would go on to affiliate with SATA started to treat TB sufferers at a refugee camp. After its founding in October 1938, SATA established a more permanent facility, which had 100 beds devoted entirely to charity cases (U38-1-191).[20] This Tuberculosis Hospital had 20 staff: seven volunteers (including two doctors and two registered nurses) and 13 paid staff (including three doctors, seven nurses, a technician, and a pharmacist). Its facilities included an operating room, lab, X-ray, pharmacy, kitchen, dorm for staff, and three wards. The hospital had room for more beds; however, SATA did not initially own enough beds to expand. SATA acquired them in part by asking donors to sponsor beds (SMA: U38-1-191[2]). The number of beds in SATA's Tuberculosis Hospital quickly expanded to 200 and 220. In SATA's *Second Annual Report*, Huizenga noted that the hospital had 230 beds, including a children's ward with 52 (SMA U38-1-191). Given their vulnerability to disease and their high likelihood of recovering, children attracted donor attention. As Margaret Tillman argues, "Emotionally and financially, children represented the best return on investment for philanthropists" (2018: 96). Donors to the Tuberculosis Hospital included companies, nonprofit organizations, and individuals. By October 1940, 85 of the 230 beds at the hospital were endowed: 50 by China Child Welfare, a New York–based nonprofit, 30 by the Shanghai International Red Cross, and another 5 by private donors. The hospital further had an outpatient clinic and pneumothorax therapy.

SATA also had a self-sustaining facility for paying patients, which was highlighted at the beginning of this chapter. On January 1, 1939, the Second Red Cross Refugee Treatment Hospital became affiliated with SATA and was renamed the Shanghai Hospital.[21] When SATA first took over the facility, it had

---

20. Lee S. Huizenga, 1939, "Report of the Tuberculosis Hospital," in *SATA's First Annual Report* (SMA: U38-1-191). The Tuberculosis Hospital was located in western Shanghai, in buildings owned by Academia Sinica, near East China Normal University, and next to St. Luke's Hospital. The Tuberculosis Hospital actually received its water supply from St. Luke's (SMA: U1-16-2663).

21. The facility was at the site of the former Linsheng (霖生) Hospital at 190 Yueyang Road.

Figure 2.1: SATA's Shanghai Hospital

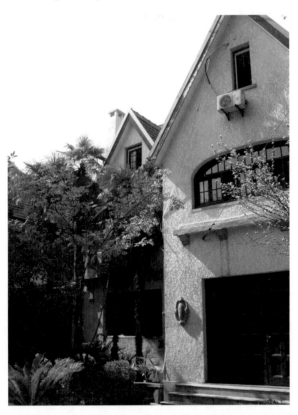

Built in 1920, this site served as Linsheng Hospital and a refugee treatment hospital before its affiliation with SATA from January 1938 to June 1941. It then became a private hospital. It was nationalized in 1956 and became the Xuhui District Tuberculosis Prevention and Treatment Clinic in 1958. Photo by the author.

6 beds for first-class patients, 14 for second-class patients, and a ward for third-class patients, but initially no beds for them. By the end of 1939, the Shanghai Hospital acquired 40 beds for the semi-charitable, third-class ward, where patients paid approximately half of their costs (SMA U38-5-1625, SMA U38-1-191[2]). Because the facility already had a number of hospitalized patients when it began its relationship with SATA in 1939, not all patients were TB sufferers. In fact, in 1939, only 213 of patients hospitalized at any point during the year had TB; 380 did not (SMA: U38-5-1625).[22]

---

22. *First Annual Report of the Shanghai Hospital of the SATA, Jan 1, 1939–Dec 31, 1939* (in SMA: U38-5-1625).

An Unrealized Vision of Health and Tuberculosis Control   67

The paying patients received more attentive care than did those in the charity hospital. Despite the fact the Shanghai Hospital had fewer than one-third the number of beds at SATA's Tuberculosis Hospital, the Shanghai Hospital's staff, at 34, was larger, including four doctors, an intern, 11 nurses, 11 nurse aids, a pharmacist, a lab technician, and five business staff.[23] Consequently, the time that medical staff could devote to each individual patient was almost certainly longer than at the Tuberculosis Hospital. The Shanghai Hospital also provided clinical training for students from nearby medical colleges. In October 1940, the hospital was training four medical students, two interns, seven nursing students, and two pharmacy students from a local medical college (SMA U1-16-2663 and U38-1-191), thus contributing to a priority of national health reconstruction.

SATA's two facilities, the Tuberculosis and Shanghai Hospitals, increased the number of TB beds in Shanghai by 290—a more than 50 percent rise from the 529 found in the January 1939 survey—but demand still far outstripped supply. In meetings and publications, Tuberculosis Hospital supervisor, Dr. Lee S. Huizenga, emphasized that these beds were always full. For instance, in a December 1, 1939, funding appeal to the French administration, Dr. Huizenga stated that 1,530 patients had already been cared for, but "the cry for more beds is so great that we could without doubt double this amount for destitute TB patients if we had the resources" (SMA U38-1-191). In 1940, the superintendent of the Shanghai Hospital similarly lamented, "A number of patients had to be turned away daily" (SMA U38-1-191).[24]

SATA continued to struggle for resources as it made good on its commitment to offer treatment to patients throughout 1940–1942. It did this by running a successful fundraising campaign and emphasizing the role of outpatient clinics. SATA's Hospital Building and Equipment Fund Campaign lasted from November 15, 1941, to February 28, 1942. The campaign involved widespread publicity based on in-kind and other donations, including free advertising at 25 theaters; 30,000 appeal letters and 10,000 illustrated folders in Chinese printed by the *China Press*; and 30,000 Chinese posters, 12,000 appeal letters in English, and 4,000 illustrated folders in English printed by the Post-Mercury Company. The successful campaign raised more than CN$1 million, more than two-and-a-half times the organization's total hospital expenses in the four previous years. This allowed SATA to purchase the former Municipal Council Sanatorium and move the Tuberculosis Hospital to the site and to found a second semi-charitable

---

23. There was actually a disconnect between SATA's charitable mission and the fact that this hospital was self-sustaining. When the hospital did turn a profit in June 1942, its staff elected to split from SATA rather than invest these profits back into the facility or SATA itself (Core 2019).

24. "Report of the Shanghai Hospital," presented in SATA's *Second Annual Report* (SMA U38-1-191).

TB hospital (SMA U1-16-2660 and U38-1-192).[25] In addition to buildings, SATA prioritized training nurses and specialists, who kept up with the latest developments in TB control. The campaign also helped SATA acquire X-ray and operation equipment and to open outpatient clinics at all hospitals. This final emphasis on outpatient clinics allowed SATA to extend its reach, particularly in 1941–1942. In the four years between October 1, 1938, and September 30, 1942, SATA had 3,000 more outpatient visits (13,952) than the number of inpatients treated (10,882) (SATA 1942). SATA's growing emphasis on free outpatient treatment is evident from the increase in outpatient visits—from 1,729 in 1939 to 6,557 in 1941.

Despite the many efforts to develop and staff TB treatment facilities, there were several problems. Most hospitalized TB sufferers did not receive any type of treatment until their disease had progressed to an advanced stage. This meant that they required longer, more costly treatment, with reduced chance for success. Indeed, the aggregate data from SATA's first four years look bleak: of 10,882 admitted patients, only 2,549 were discharged, and 1,314 of these discharged patients (52.61 percent) died. These numbers speak to the many challenges of combatting a widespread infectious disease in a situation of resource scarcity. Disaggregating the data by facility suggests differential treatment success based on patient background. For instance, in 1939, more TB patients were discharged from the Shanghai Hospital with "improved," "arrested," or "apparently arrested" disease than died from the disease. However, at the Tuberculosis Hospital that same year, twice as many patients died from the disease as were discharged in "apparently arrested" or "improved" condition (SMA U38-1-191; Core 2014). Better chances for survival among patients at the Shanghai Hospital were most likely because they were paying patients with better access to resources than the charity patients. The Shanghai Hospital patients' backgrounds allowed them better access to nutritious food and health care throughout their lives. By contrast, many patients at the Tuberculosis Hospital delayed seeking care until it was too late.

Currency fluctuations and rising costs during the war were an additional challenge to TB treatment. For instance, when International Settlement residents inquired about the status of the closed Municipal Council Sanatorium in local daily newspapers in 1940, the annual cost for reopening was estimated to be twice the prewar cost (SMA: U1-16-654). SATA's Tuberculosis Hospital reports indicate that the cost of operation more than doubled between late 1939 and

---

25. *SATA Bulletin* 1, no. 5 (May 31, 1942) and nos. 6/7 (June–July 1942) in SMA U1-16-2660. *SATA Bulletin* 1, nos. 10–12 (October–December 1942) in SMA U38-1-192. The second (semi-charitable) tuberculosis hospital made up for the loss of the Shanghai Hospital, when staff at this facility severed their relationship with SATA on July 1, 1942 (Core 2019).

An Unrealized Vision of Health and Tuberculosis Control

early 1940, only to stabilize somewhat during the following year (SMA: U38-1-191).[26] Price fluctuations of the goods required for operation added urgency to SATA's pleas for funding both from government and private sources. SATA's application for aid from the French Municipal Council on October 3, 1940, noted that costs for food at the Tuberculosis Hospital in 1940 outweighed the total expenses from October 1938 to August 1939 (SMA: U1-16-2662, U38-1-191[1], U38-5-1625). In 1941, SATA representatives mentioned the soaring cost of food in their request to waive taxes and increase grant-in-aid from the FMC; food costs made up more than half the budget for the Tuberculosis Hospital for that year (SMA U1-16-2662; SMA U38-1-191).

To alleviate inflationary pressures, SATA sought in-kind donations of items for its hospitals—foodstuffs, linens, and even hospital equipment. The collaborationist government's seizure of borrowed equipment and furniture from the Shanghai Hospital, mentioned at the beginning of this chapter, highlights the danger of relying on long-term, in-kind loans of equipment. In other cases, donations supported day-to-day needs. SATA's *Quarterly Report* for June to August 1941 detailed SATA's receipt of 10 tons of rice, eight cases of powdered milk, and three tons of soft coal (SMA: U1-16-2663). Receipt of these items helped to control room and board expenses, at least for that year. As the war progressed, the funding situation became more dire in 1942–1943. SATA's Medical Committee reported on expenses through February 1943 at a Standing Committee meeting on May 5, 1943, stating, "When the *cost of everything*, particularly of food and other necessities of life, has risen to an unprecedented level, extended hospitalization of free patients becomes an unbearable burden to the institution" (SMA R50-1-140; SMA U1-16-2661, emphasis in the original). At the same meeting, SATA proudly reported that all of it funding in 1942 had come from local sources, which signaled that the organization was moving beyond a colonial model, where much of its financial support had come from foreign governments and donors.

Archival records on TB control for the final two years of the war with the Japanese, 1943–1945, are not as complete as those for the previous years; however, there is some evidence that SATA and other organizations continued their work. By 1943, Western governments had relinquished their control over the treaty ports, and the Japanese had taken charge of the SMC, including the health department. On August 16, 1943, the Municipal Council secretary general, K. Takagi, authorized a CN$55,000 grant-in-aid for SATA, which allowed it to continue to provide services to TB sufferers in 1944.

Separating TB sufferers from the general public was a concern for decades prior to the 1943 discovery of streptomycin, and various actors in

---

26. Oct. 1938 to Feb 1941 *Report of the Tuberculosis Hospital.*

Shanghai—public, private, and nonprofit—sought to do this. This section has highlighted efforts to make beds available to the poor to partially correct the previous imbalance in who received hospital care. To reduce the strain on resources, SATA and other institutions in Shanghai promoted pneumothorax as well as outpatient treatment. Unfortunately, neither SATA nor the governments addressed the underlying factors contributing to TB infection.

A New Era of TB Control, 1946–1949

The postwar era ushered in a new period of optimism in the fight against diseases, both internationally and in China. As the world reorganized into capitalist and communist geopolitical camps, multilateral organizations, including the World Health Organization (WHO) also formed. Demonstrating success with health initiatives became one strategy of Cold War rivalry. China was also influenced by both the optimism and the rivalry. As the Japanese Occupation was coming to an end, the GMD began to explore models for providing health care to the entire population. Despite growing domestic conflict with the Communists, the GMD concluded that the Soviet Union's free health-care system might be a model to emulate (Gao 2014). In the postwar years, attempts were certainly made to make TB control more widely available.

Following the Japanese Occupation of Shanghai, more widespread and sustained efforts by the Chinese government focused on TB prevention. In 1946, Wu Shaoqing (吴绍青, 1895–1980), professor at Shanghai Medical College and director of the Pulmonary Department at the Zhongshan Hospital, led the formation of the Shanghai Coordinating Committee for Tuberculosis Control from 12 civic and medical bodies including SATA and the Shanghai Medical College (SMA Q400-1-4053). This committee's efforts signaled a new commitment to bringing TB control to the grassroots population. In the postwar years, the Coordinating Committee helped to step up prevention efforts. In a 1947 article, Wu wrote, "Tuberculosis is cruel because we don't pay attention to health education. . . . When promoting health education, TB should be the first priority (1931)." Wu's characterization gives no credit to the preventive education attempts of the GMD government or SATA, but his points about the need to prioritize TB education was spot on.

Wu was particularly concerned with education as a means of making the people aware of symptoms so they would not wait until it was too late to report to treatment facilities, a problem that had contributed to high mortality and morbidity in SATA's Tuberculosis Hospital. Wu thought education was the only way to improve upon this situation. To this end, schools and other workplaces became the target of educational campaigns. On June 29, 1947, Wu Shaoqing led 23 universities and 70 middle schools—more than 10,000 people—to form

An Unrealized Vision of Health and Tuberculosis Control 71

more than 1,000 small groups to expand the anti-TB movement in schools (CMA 1997). At SATA's ninth annual meeting, on April 16, 1948, the Publicity Committee also reported that in 1947, a Seventh-day Adventist minister and recovered TB patient lectured in factories and schools: "103 middle schools were visited with an audience of approximately 52,500 students" (SMA Q199-20-43). Thus, in the postwar era, organizations finally started to make good on GMD intentions regarding preventive health. This is the first evidence of wide-scale prevention efforts that would be developed on a much larger scale in work units after the 1949 Communist victory.

The Coordinating Committee also engaged in other TB control activities that would become more widespread in the following decades. As the BCG vaccine and antibiotics came into widespread distribution and use internationally in the 1940s, there was great optimism that TB would finally be conquered (Raviglione and Pio 2002; McMillen and Brimnes 2010). BCG had not been among the therapies NATAC and SATA had promoted; however, Shanghai developed better vaccination capacity and continued to work in this area during the war. Between 1946 and 1949, "hundreds of thousands of residents received vaccines against" infectious diseases, including cholera, smallpox, typhoid, and diphtheria (Henriot 2016: 31). Expanded vaccination programs allowed the Coordinating Committee for TB Control to promote BCG inoculations. The number of BCG shots was far fewer than cholera or smallpox immunizations, but the committee's annual report for 1947 stated that 740 children received BCG in the previous year. This was nearly 10 percent of the total BCG shots estimated to have been given in Shanghai prior to 1948 (Brazelton 2019a).

Likewise, active case finding (ACF) became more widespread in Shanghai, as it was elsewhere in the world at this time. Previously, case finding had been done only on a limited basis. SATA's 1939 survey of TB facilities noted available X-ray equipment, but during the Japanese Occupation, ACF was largely not conducted owing to lack of treatment facilities for those discovered to have TB. After the war, the Hongqiao Sanatorium conducted 3,224 TB-related checkups in the first half of 1946. Of persons who received checkups, 795, or 24.66 percent, were found to have TB, an astounding statistic that suggested a backlog of unidentified cases and a need for further widespread testing. Of those with TB, 582 (or 73.21 percent) were between the ages of 10 and 33 (CMA 1997), indicating high prevalence, particularly among children and young adults. The Coordinating Committee for TB Control also did chest X-rays and group health checks after the war, including chest X-rays on 6,425 people in October through December 1947 (SMA Q400-1-4053). SATA also prioritized this work. The American Committee of SATA donated X-ray equipment so a lighter machine the organization already owned could be mounted on a donated Chevy truck to increase

72   *Tuberculosis Control and Institutional Change in Shanghai*

case-finding capacity (SMA Q199-20-43). This would become an important part of SATA's work after it was nationalized in the 1950s.

In the final years of the 1940s, the Coordinating Committee developed a plan for reaching everyone in TB control. In 1947, Wu wrote, "If everyone gets a chest X-ray, infected persons are treated and their contacts are traced, this will prevent the spread of the disease. If a check-up is done each year, this can protect every group's safety" (Wu 1947: 31). Wu clarified his meaning of "group" in a 1949 article. "The group should be the workplace [*danwei*, 单位]. Make sure every person gets a chest X-ray . . . then separate them into treatment groups: those receiving outpatient treatment and those checked according to schedule, and then hospitalized. Another group can rest at home, but they should be separated from other family members' activities" (Wu 1949: 1). Wu's ideas would become the cornerstone of post-1949 efforts to extend anti-TB work to a larger proportion of the population.

The Shanghai Coordinating Committee for Tuberculosis Control also opened a TB clinical center at the site of the Chinese First Red Cross Hospital's former TB outpatient clinic on March 10, 1947.[27] This clinic received 11,750 patient visits in the remaining months of 1947. The Coordinating Committee also helped to recover the Chengzhong Hospital, which reopened on April 20, 1947, with 74 beds, a 90 percent occupancy rate, and plans to expand to 200 beds (SMA Q400-1-4053). In 1949, Wu Shaoqing reported that TB treatment rooms were being added to general hospital wards and sanatoria founded to receive TB sufferers. At the time of the Communist victory in October 1949, the city had 841 designated TB sick beds and 58 specialists (CMA 1997). These beds were located in 41 facilities, including 13 governmental, 11 collective, and 17 private. Although certainly an improvement upon the number of beds available in 1939, this number was far too few for the estimated number of cases in the city. TB in China was as severe as anywhere in the world; however, Wu claimed China had only one sick bed per every 4 million people, compared to the United States and Europe, where there was one sick bed for every 1,000 people (Wu 1949). It is impossible to verify these statistics; however, the situation was dire. As the following two chapters will illustrate, efforts to control TB became more comprehensive in the 1950s.

Conclusion

Disease control was an issue of national pride. The 1928–1937 National Reconstruction Program aimed to cure China's image as the "sick man of Asia" but was not fully implemented owing to lack of resources to build and

---

27. Today, this site is part of Huashan Hospital.

staff infrastructure. At the time, a great deal of governmental funds went to the military, to wage war against the Japanese and manage internal conflicts with regional warlords and Communists. This limited resources that could be expended on developing the infrastructure and the organizational capacity necessary for extending TB control to the wider population and truly achieving the GMD vision for health.

Some public health campaigns were carried out. Yet TB prevention campaigns largely missed the working poor, such as dock workers and other semi-employed individuals whose living conditions made them most susceptible to disease. Many educational campaigns aimed to raise awareness of TB control efforts among the middle class and potential donors to nonprofit organizations. Certainly, having funds available to treat TB patients is an extremely important part of TB control; however, pitching TB control programs to persons whose living conditions made them most susceptible to the disease is what is ultimately necessary for prevention. The Japanese Occupation of Shanghai further provided challenges to TB control because it prompted problems with displaced refugees, damaged facilities, and skyrocketing prices for the items used in TB wards. A public health model had not yet been developed to actively engage a large proportion of the population, particularly those with little education or unstable work. The state had the will and intention but not yet the institutional means to carry out effective public health work. Globally, great strides in TB medicines were made during the World War II and in the years immediately following. Following the war, SATA recovered, and the Coordinating Committee for Tuberculosis Control made greater efforts to extend TB control to the grassroots level. The next two chapters will demonstrate the deepening of these efforts after 1949.

Part II

Work-Unit Era, 1950–1992

3

Embracing a New Scientific Health Image in the Work Unit, 1950–1957

Case-finding work, which the Shanghai Coordinating Committee for Tuberculosis Control began to emphasize in the postwar years, became much more systematic and widespread during the early Mao years. For example, in July 1953, 3,063 workers at the Fifth National Cotton Factory received chest X-rays (Song 1953). One hundred and one workers were found to have active but mild cases of TB. In September 1953, the factory set up a TB infirmary (自办疗养所) where 47 of the patients rested all the time and 54 rested part time (Chen and Sun 1954). After two months, 23 patients were able to return to their positions at work, and 21 patients who had been resting full time started resting just at night. In addition to treatment through rest and as necessary, antibiotics, improved nutrition was part of the treatment regimen. TB patients had four dishes at each meal: a soup, two protein dishes, and a vegetable dish.[1] After a year, 45 of the patients recovered and returned to their positions (Song and Chen 1954).

By the end of 1955, two additional health checks had been conducted at the factory (Song and Chen 1956). Rate of lost labor due to illness improved markedly during these years of targeted campaigns. For factory employees, rate of lost labor due to TB illness for October 1953 was 2.59 percent; by the end of 1955, this rate was .233 percent. By the end of 1955, 139 workers had been treated for TB: 75 using antibiotics, 52 through rest and nutrition, 7 through collapse therapy, and 5 through other operations. In 1956, 74 of these workers (53.24 percent) had recovered, 4 others had improved in condition, and 2 had worsened. While the rest were still being treated, average stay in the infirmary was shortened following the second check-up. This indicates either that treatment therapies had become

---

1. For diseases such as heart disease and hypertension, doctors recommend weight loss; however, maintaining or gaining weight has often been the goal for TB patients, which was met through the improved nutrition program at the Fifth National Cotton Factory. Of 38 patients with detailed case records, 29 gained weight (with an average increase of 3.3 kg), seven had no change in weight, and two lost half to a full kg (Chen and Sun 1954: 7).

more efficient or that cases were being discovered at an earlier stage of disease progression and were easier to treat. The Fifth National Cotton Factory and its recovered workers were held up as models for other workplaces to emulate (SMA B168-1-818). Song and Chen (1954) report that six other factories built infirmaries within a year after the Fifth National Factory's opened.

The Fifth National Cotton Factory's TB case finding and treatment experience was particularly well documented in *Shanghai Anti-TB* (上海防痨), *Anti-TB Journal* (防痨通讯), *Health News* (健康报), and archival sources. The articles about this case emphasize that recovered patients should play an active role in demonstrating that TB is treatable. The articles also contain some slightly exaggerated propaganda about patients receiving medical care—"under the leadership of the CCP and Mao, they could achieve happiness"—but articles also made the practical suggestion that recovered workers' bodies were the best propaganda (Song and Chen 1954). Clearly, workers who did not have access to treatment facilities before 1950 would have been elated, and their improved health could be used as evidence that new state policies were effective.

Health is socially constructed, and norms are reinforced through symbols and rituals. Envisioning and attempting to actualize a new health image was part of the state-led reimaging that happened during the early Mao era, 1950–1957. Recent scholarship has examined how the new Chinese state used institutions and imagery to mobilize workers to adopt new cultural and political norms in the 1950s (Perry 2002; Hung 2011, 2021; D. Y. Ho 2017; Xiao and Li 2020). This chapter contributes to the scholarship on the early Mao years by demonstrating how pervasive new institutions in urban areas attempted to create and reinforce norms of improved sanitation and infectious disease control. In the early 1950s, work units became a chief organization involved in health promotion and became the grassroots implementation points for tuberculosis control, including preventive programming, identifying active cases of disease, and providing treatment, often with new antibiotics and in isolated spaces, such as the TB infirmary at the Fifth National Cotton Factory. This chapter provides an overview of the creation of the work-unit system and how it helped to stabilize population. Work units then became grassroots facilities for gathering information about the population. The analysis then turns to disease prevention, monitoring, and treatment. The state enacted prevention in several ways: by making general quality-of-life improvements, through vaccination campaigns, and through widespread health education. As part of this education, images and slogans were plastered on the walls of schools and workplaces. Constituents were then expected to emulate these images. Various forms of health monitoring—including documenting participation in health campaigns and tuberculosis case finding—followed directly from this. The final step to actualizing this new health image was commitment to cover the cost of treatment, which became a widespread norm during this era. Because TB control was relatively successful, disease control became part of the regimen that the Communist government used to demonstrate the efficacy of socialism. Health promotion and provision became aligned with economic development and ultimately helped to promote political stability.

Creation of the Work-Unit System, 1950–1957

On October 1, 1949, the decades of fighting between the Guomindang and the Communists came to an end when the Communists seized control of the Chinese mainland and the GMD fled to Taiwan. In the subsequent era of stability, the Communist government created a strong central state and began to socialize the economy. The government adopted the paradigm of socialist planning and built the institutions necessary to realize it. Key among these institutions was the work unit. The government created the work-unit system as it took over private enterprises, GMD state enterprises, banks, government offices, schools, hospitals, and other health organizations, such as the Shanghai Anti-Tuberculosis Association.[2] In urban areas, the system was established in three steps before 1957. First, the government compelled capitalists, such as the owners of cotton mills, to turn over their firms. Second, the government organized petty capitalists—dock workers, rickshaw pullers, noodle sellers, bicycle mechanics, barbers, and so on—into collective enterprises. Finally, the government encouraged housewives and other unemployed persons to pool their talents and resources and establish small factories and workshops within their neighborhoods (Whyte and Parish 1984). As the government hired unemployed intellectuals to be teachers and administrators in secondary schools, schools also expanded starting in 1950 (U 2007). Thereafter, all urban residents were expected to be members of one of these units, from the time they graduated from high school or college until they died.

In practice, this system was not created in a neat process, nor was full employment ever achieved. The takeover of organizations was part of a shift in Communist policies toward cities, and Shanghai had a special, symbolic place in it. The central government needed the Communist takeover of Shanghai and other key cities to succeed in order to legitimate its rule. Securing Shanghai was important politically, economically, and culturally; and the state took over enterprises in each of these realms with varying degrees of success. In the economic realm, factories would bring in revenue for the state, but they also had symbolic significance, since the worker was considered the vanguard of the revolution. In

---

2. In rural areas, a similar system would be established through the process of agricultural collectivization between 1950 and 1957; however, the types of welfare provided in rural areas were much less complete than those in urban areas.

the first years after the Communist takeover, the participation of former enterprise owners was in flux and negotiated. A culture of accommodation arose in which some groups (such as capitalists) collaborated in their own demise, but individuals also had room to maneuver (Strauss 2006; Brown and Pickowicz 2012; Howlett 2013). The creation of new cultural norms was a concern of not just economic production units but also entertainment venues. In the cultural realm, organizations such as publishers, radio stations, cinemas, and cultural palaces could help to propagate and reinforce new norms, including health norms (Johnson 2015; J. Li 2020; Xiao and Li 2020; Hung 2021).

Private facilities were also nationalized and infrastructure expanded in the health sector among organizations, such as SATA, and formerly private hospitals. For instance, in February 1956, the Private Shanghai Hospital became the Public Shanghai Hospital when it was nationalized. This facility had been SATA's Shanghai Hospital from January 1939 to June 1942. After severing its relationship with SATA, it became profit oriented from 1944 until 1956. In the 1950s, it underwent two additional transformations: it was nationalized in 1956, and it became the Xuhui District Tuberculosis Prevention and Treatment Clinic in 1958 (Mei, Zhong, and Wang 1991; Provider 18). Chapter 4 further examines how this venue became a key participant in the TB control network after 1958. This clinic was only one example of the expansive state infrastructure for health developed during this period, which helped achieve higher levels of employment, as well as health benefit provision.

While the work-unit system never succeeded in bringing all urban residents into its orb, work units, nevertheless, became the heart of economic and social life in urban areas. Under the planned economy, the government centrally set production targets and took responsibility for the distribution of goods and services. Work units were the distribution points and became known as their members' "iron rice bowl" (铁饭碗), a term that emphasizes the unbreakable link between workers and the entitlements provided through places of employment. In addition to salaries, work units distributed food coupons, subsidized cafeterias and housing, managed pensions, and provided daycare or schooling for workers' children (Lü and Perry 1997). Indeed, work unit provisions went well beyond the economic benefits of Western workplaces. On the flip side of these generous provisions, however, work units encroached on many areas of life, becoming inescapable in the social realm.

In the social realm, work units controlled both reproduction and mobility, often cutting their members off from wider society. Work units took responsibility for functions formerly carried out in the family, including approval of marriages and provision of family planning. The work-unit system was part of a broad array of new institutions, including household registration (*hukou*) and food-rationing systems that effectively curbed migration. Other scholars have pointed out that these institutions sought to divide the population through exclusion and control (Y. Bian 1994; F.-L. Wang 2005; Brown 2012). Work units controlled their members' dossiers, which minimized social mobility. While work units became total institutions—inescapable places controlling nearly all aspects of life—the members of these urban institutions were also relatively privileged.[3] Work-unit provisions helped to solidify the unequal dichotomy set up through the household registration system, which ensured that urban workers did not have to worry where their next meal was coming from. Persons who worked the land in rural areas were not nearly so lucky—they were required to produce enough grain both for their families and to support urban workers (Lü and Perry 1997; Brown 2012).

Given that it was a total institution that was coercive at times, the work-unit system worked very well for controlling disease. In the realm of health, the CCP built the work unit into an effective link between individuals and public health and medical infrastructure. Work units provided medical insurance, primary care, and the channel into the medical system for workers. To do this, the system expanded upon the GMD efforts to found workplace clinics and train health personnel to work in them (M. L. Bian 2005). Larger work units had attached hospitals or clinics. The workplace became the implementation point for both general public health programs and TB control campaigns that involved employees and their families in the health system. Work units socialized their members to adopt new health behavior and practices and put systems in place to police health behaviors and ensure compliance.

Population Control and TB Control in Shanghai

In Shanghai, creation of the work-unit system helped to stabilize the population. While the precise population of the metropolis at the time of the Communist takeover is unknown, it was certainly around 5 million. Drawing upon documentation from the Shanghai Municipal Archives, Jonathan Howlett notes that at the end of 1948, Shanghai's population was 5.44 million, with 420,000 industrial workers employed in 12,500 factories, including 45 percent of the nation's textile manufacturers (2013). Christian Henriot notes that population estimates varied by source and year. In 1947 the municipal police recorded 4.2 million residents; however, other scholars have retrospectively claimed a population of 5.5 million in 1949 (Henriot 2016: 15). After the Communist takeover, many poor people were pushed out of urban areas, resulting in a 1950 population

---

3. Goffman defined the total institution as a "place of residence and work where a large number of like situated individuals, cut off from the wider society for an appreciable period of time, together led an enclosed, formerly administered round of life" (Goffman 1961: xiii).

of around 4.8 million; but poverty in the countryside pushed 400,000 into the city by June 1951 (J. Y. Chen 2012; Henriot 2016). Other scholars concur that estimating an exact population was difficult because approximately 85 percent of urban residents were born outside the city (Feng, Zuo, and Ruan 2002). The 1950–1957 period was one of large-scale in- and out-migration, with in-migration far exceeding out-migration (Gui and Liu 1992). Unsurprisingly, scholarly accounts differ regarding the size of the population in 1953: some put it at 5.35 million in urban areas, others claim it was 6.2 million (Zhu 2008; Henriot 2016). In 1958, Shanghai expanded its boundaries to include 10 counties that were previously part of neighboring Jiangsu and Zhejiang Provinces (Zhu 2008).[4] After the work-unit system was in place, Shanghai's population growth decelerated, then stagnated. Between the 1964 and 1982 censuses, it averaged only 0.5 percent per year—from 10.82 million to 11.86 million.

Shanghai's large population was, by no means, homogenous. City residents came from a host of different backgrounds. Some were new to the city; other families had been there for decades. Some had education or skills; others lacked skills but were still drawn to opportunities in the city. Understandings of health and the body were also heterogeneous and changing in this period. Despite the differing understanding of disease, both new and old residents likely agreed that dying from TB was not a good thing. Thus, during the early 1950s, the state set about socializing urban residents to participate in—or at least not to openly resist—state encroachment into the realm of bodily matters. TB control became an area where the state eventually created a new socially constructed reality. As Chapter 4 emphasizes, this process was never complete; however, enough medical advances were made available to a large enough portion of the population to have a lasting impact on TB.

Given the difficulties in estimating the total population of Shanghai, determining accurate TB morbidity and mortality is even more difficult. TB remained the most widespread and deadliest urban infectious disease when the Chinese Communist Party came to power in 1949. Based on the best data we have, during the 1950s, TB mortality rates in Shanghai fell dramatically from 208 deaths per 100,000 in 1951 to 31 deaths per 100,000 in 1965 (Sun 1981; Figure 3.1). Before 1956, TB was the leading cause of death in the city; by 1983, just 27 years later, it fell to the tenth leading cause (CMA 1997). How was this decline in TB achieved and sustained?

Declining TB was, undoubtedly, the result of a combination of factors, including steady employment, a stable food supply, and better overall living conditions, as well as medical advances that did not exist before the Japanese

---

4. Ash (1981) estimates that if these counties had already been part of Shanghai, the city's population would have been 7 million in 1949 and almost 10 million in 1957.

Embracing a New Scientific Health Image 83

Figure 3.1: Shanghai's tuberculosis mortality rates

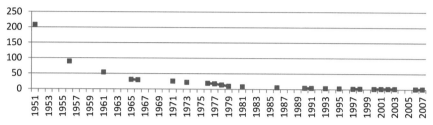

Sources: Mortality rates for 1950–1979 are from Sun (1981). Post-1980 mortality rates are from Shanghai yearbooks.

Occupation. It was convenient for the Communist state that effective antibiotics against TB were discovered at the same time as state consolidation occurred. Some of the medical advances, such as immunizations, widescale case finding, and effective antibiotics, were game changers, but medical advances cannot reach the population without an effective distribution system and popular acceptance of these advances, whether willingly or through coercion. The work-unit system allowed for delivery of both quality-of-life and medical improvements. The following sections examine the process through which the state socialized and at times, coerced the population to adopt health interventions at the grassroots level.

Invigorating Prevention Efforts

Prevention of infectious disease was a cornerstone of the Communist health model, both in China and in other areas of the world. China adopted several aspects of the Soviet model, including articulating the importance of strong and healthy workers, establishing more than 600 prevention and treatment stations nationwide, and training medical and sanitation workers at the local level (Michaels 2003; Gao 2014). Tuberculosis control campaigns, such as the one in the Fifth National Cotton Factory, encouraged workplace leaders to assimilate the Soviet experience, while also considering local conditions (Song 1954). Chinese urban and rural areas developed teams to implement preventive programming, often on a mass scale (M.-s. Chen 2001; Gross and Fan 2014; Gross 2016; Zhou 2020). In 1950, Shanghai's Health Bureau established 21,000 public health groups (卫生小组) to implement citywide health movements (Henriot 2016: 21). Prevention activities included both direct disease control efforts, such as widespread BCG inoculations and education about disease transmission means and symptoms, and indirect efforts that aimed to improve health more generally. Both general and specific prevention programs included a plethora of visual materials understandable to semiliterate members of the public.

The 1950s prevention programs also included the public in the Patriotic Hygiene Campaign (爱国卫生运动), which linked prevention to production. The Communist government launched the campaign in 1952. It was patriotic, first, in that it was directed against the perceived threat of US germ warfare on the Korean Peninsula and in Manchuria (Rogaski 2002, 2022). Second, it was designed to improve the health of the Chinese people—making them strong and boosting their productive capacity so that China's output of steel and other heavy industrial products could compete with the United States and England. The campaign was run by a committee aligned with the Ministry of Health (Patriotic Hygiene Committee 1953). It urged mass mobilization of various societal groups, including health professionals, and as Wayne Soon notes, such campaigns "artificially fostered a sense of wartime urgency," allowing for the expansion of biomedicine and public health programs (Soon 2020: 203). Activities dedicated to eliminating specific diseases—such as TB and schistosomiasis—came under the umbrella of the Patriotic Hygiene Campaign, and the work unit became the implementation point for many of these efforts.

By assuming responsibility for many goods and services that the family had previously provided, the 1950s workplace improved the standard of living and general health. Housing was among the most important services the work unit provided. Housing allocation itself varied greatly by work unit and did not always include a private kitchen or bathroom. The limited housing stock in Shanghai and many other cities often precluded married adults leaving their parents' home. Nevertheless, housing provision was designed to eliminate crowded shantytowns, and from the standpoint of infectious disease control, this meant fewer opportunities for disease transmission. Work units also provided cafeterias with simple, hot meals three times a day and access to facilities for bathing.[5] As mentioned in the chapter opening, factories with TB infirmaries provided extra nutrition for those recovering from TB. Having access to nutritious meals and hygiene facilities improved worker health and mitigated the proximate and distal causes of TB infection and disease progression.

Other quality-of-life improvements in the 1950s included shortening working hours and providing recreational facilities. Workplaces began to scale back the number of working hours from the 12-hour day, six days per week that pre-1949 capitalist factories required (Murphey 1953; G. Zhang 1954;

---

5. Some employees of the Chinese work units where I was based in 1998–2002 still showered at their workplace, rather than at home.

Honig 1986). Having time to rest improved workers' health, as did making use of communal recreation facilities. Larger work units featured recreation halls and installed loudspeakers that blasted news, music, and morning exercise instructions (J. Li 2020).[6] Smaller work units, such as restaurants, department stores, and transportation stations, often still required workers to participate in morning exercises (Brownell 1995). In these ways, work units improved workers' general living conditions as proposed but not fully realized by the National Health Reconstruction program.

In terms of direct disease prevention, promotion of vaccines, including BCG, was one of the earliest parts of Communist-era prevention efforts (Henriot 2016; Brazelton 2019a, 2019b). After its founding in 1948, the newly formed World Health Organization also widely promoted BCG. Thus, China's widespread efforts were in line with international recommendations, despite its exclusion from the WHO. On January 16, 1950, the *People's Daily* (人民日报) reported that the Ministry of Health (promoted free BCG vaccination for children under five, young workers, students, and soldiers. The article encouraged families to bring young children to be immunized (Zhi 1950). Workplaces and school health personnel ran free immunization clinics for young workers and students.

Archival data suggests that BCG vaccination occurred on a massive scale. According to the work report of the Shanghai Municipal Patriotic Hygiene Campaign, 53,791 persons received the BCG vaccine during the first 10 months of 1952 (SMA B242-1-535-60). In 1953, 20,000 people took BCG orally, and 67,437 received injections in Shanghai (CATA 1954). During the collectivization of industry, schools, and hospitals, the proportion of infants immunized in Shanghai increased even more dramatically, from under 10 percent in 1953 to nearly 80 percent in 1959 (SMA B242-1-1510; Core 2014). This emphasis on vaccination built upon a wider push for scientific development, directed both toward bodies and into the workplace. People were asked to be active members of this process.

Prevention was also done through pervasive education programs. Preventive education in the workplace included lectures and slide shows by health professionals or trained workers and widespread visual imagery, including exhibits and posters. Other scholars have examined how visual displays were used to create and reinforce new norms, as resocialization of the population occurred after 1949. For example, Denise Ho examines how exhibits became "a form of participatory propaganda," sparking political awakening and motivating participation

---

6. During a semester studying abroad in 1995, I was awakened each morning by the Nankai University loudspeaker announcements, including counts for repetitions of morning exercises. This practice has continued on university campuses and workplaces well into the twenty-first century.

in Shanghai's neighborhoods (2017: 13). Likewise, Chang-tai Hung examines how visual imagery was manipulated for propaganda in urban spaces where the new state sought to consolidate control of the nation's capital, including publishers, newspapers, cultural palaces, and parks (2011, 2021). As other scholars have demonstrated, science, medicine, and disease control were also brought into the wheelhouse of the state propaganda machine (Gross 2016; Schmalzer 2016). Science and health content featured among the displays in workplaces—including factories, schools, press offices, and cultural palaces—as the state sought to create a new reality.

Shanghai's workplaces and alleyways became a canvas for both general and disease-specific health programming. Posters and other public health materials adorned the workshop and classroom walls and appeared in displays near the factory gates. One exhibit, which was held in 1953–1954, included a series of thirty 15 × 20-inch posters. Five thousand copies of each poster were printed, and they were taken to workplaces, including factories, schools, and government offices throughout Shanghai.[7] Workers and students would have passed these posters daily as they entered their work unit, so the posters would have served as a constant visual reminder of the new health norm that government affiliates, such as SATA and work-unit health officers, aimed to create.[8] Some of the posters even depict posters within their images, illustrating how campaigns should be conducted. The content of 1950s TB prevention materials includes medical knowledge and information about TB transmission and disease symptoms. Figure 3.2 is a poster from the 1953–1954 campaign explaining respiratory routes of transmission (SATA 1953–1954). Information on the symptoms of TB in other posters encouraged common people to seek medical attention. Public health materials also advised workers to go to their workplace clinics upon recognizing these symptoms.

Widespread educational outreach directed toward workers, students, and soldiers was a hallmark of preventive programs, including anti-TB work, during the early Mao era (M.-s. Chen 2001; Bu 2017). The Shanghai Anti-Tuberculosis Association's 1952 *Annual Report* lists the type and place of health education sessions, including the approximate number of persons who attended those programs. That year, anti-TB lectures were held in 23 work units, including 12 schools and seven factories (SATA 1953a; Core 2014). TB prevention slide shows were also held in 6 of those schools and one factory. Counts of the type of public health outreach being done over seven years, from 1949 to 1955, were

---

7. Twenty-eight of the 30 posters are found in US National Library of Medicine's Chinese Public Health Collection.
8. Schools did not provide their pupils with salary and benefits, so it would be difficult to argue that schools were the "work units" of their pupils, but schools were the place at which the state extended its reach to children.

Figure 3.2: Respiratory disease transmission means

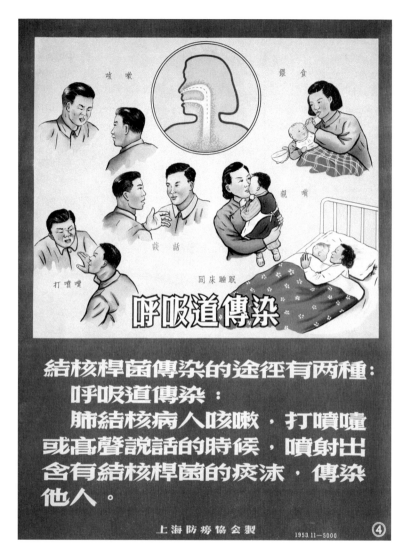

SATA 1953. Courtesy of the United States National Library of Medicine.

88   *Tuberculosis Control and Institutional Change in Shanghai*

presented at the Municipal Anti-TB Work Representative Meeting on November 25, 1956 (SMA B168-1-818). Attended by leading doctors and public health professionals, this meeting allowed SATA to summarize what it had accomplished and plan for the future. TB prevention education continued even as the representatives met. According to a plan by the Shanghai Municipal Tuberculosis Prevention Committee, during the final three quarters of 1956, TB prevention work advanced to 79 factories, reaching 114,445 workers (SMA B242-1-194). Types of TB education materials discussed at the meeting included both lectures and slide shows, as well as an increasing number of visual media, which will be discussed below (Table 3.1).

Table 3.1: Number of persons reached in TB educational programs

	1949	1950	1951	1952	1953	1954	1955
Lectures			1,125	32,037	27,067	14,703	5,045
Slides			4,450	20,441			5,700
Fliers						44,220	26,408
Exhibits	139,000	126,000			5,200	182,000	25,061

Source: SMA B168-1-818, "1956 Shanghai Municipal Anti-TB Work Representative Meeting Documents."

It is impossible to assess the veracity of statistics regarding the number of educational programs and attendees; however, emphasis on frequent, visual displays represents a major shift in public health outreach. Scholars, such as K. C. Yip (1995), note the dearth of standardized public health materials in the 1930s. Chapter 2 demonstrated that the public health materials that did exist were intended for the literate public. In the 1950s, fliers and especially public health posters, with less text and more didactic pictures, became an important part of renewed prevention activities. Expansion of schools during the era and simplification of the written script also helped to raise literacy rates, making the text on health materials more accessible. SATA published numerous posters in 1953–1955 and held large exhibits in 1949, 1951, and 1954 (SMA B168-1-818).

The counts of attendees at lectures, slide shows, and exhibits do not indicate whether attendees actually understood materials being presented or mobilized themselves to prevent disease, but creating active involvement in health was their goal. SATA publications contain guidelines on how to mobilize workers. In a 1953 article on the early results of TB prevention work in the Fifth National Cotton Factory, Song Yandong advised that after seeing traveling anti-TB exhibits, workers should give reports in small group settings (1953). Additional health personnel were trained to bring about compliance. Specifically, the state trained a coterie of "TB prevention nurses" to lead these programs. They did not serve TB patients in hospitals; instead, they took responsibility for education and outreach (Wu 1952). Wu Shaoqing estimated that in 1952, the number of TB prevention nurses in Shanghai was no more than 12. To truly "make prevention the most important part of TB work" and allow prevention to enter the workplace and family, Wu believed at least 1,500 TB prevention nurses were needed. Accurate data on the number of nurses actually trained during the period do not exist, but when asked about how campaigns were implemented, some of my respondents confirmed that the first cohorts of prevention nurses was trained during this period (Providers 12, 16, and 17). Another interviewee who completed medical school in 1953 and used to go to factories to do anti-TB work corroborated that a participatory model was used in many workplaces. Instead of having a panel of doctors at the front of a large auditorium, health educational programs split doctors and workers into smaller groups to maximize the workers' understanding and participation (Provider 8). Certainly, not all programming allowed for interaction, but this interview and the propaganda materials themselves suggest it was an aim.

Heath images and programming were pervasive, but were they effective? To determine whether educational interventions were "successful," we would need to test people's knowledge before and after interventions. Another measure of success might be whether people's actions changed in response to campaigns. While some people undoubtedly resisted invasive measures, many learned to play the part and to embrace interventions, which led to better disease control outcomes. Health campaigns were an area for the "heightened emotional commitment" and performance, as Elizabeth Perry has highlighted in her work on 1950s mobilization (2002: 112). Many industrial workers, employees in other enterprises, and students embraced new health norms. Moreover, mechanisms to ensure compliance were formed in many workplaces, as well as residential areas. The following section turns to the mechanisms that the state enacted to monitor disease vectors, as well as direct TB case finding.

Complying with Health Interventions

Early 1950s public health efforts included two primary types of activities aimed at bringing about compliance to new health norms: monitoring by both leaders and peers, and activities aimed at early case detection, such as conducting chest X-rays. Not only government officials and work unit leaders but also workers and even children carried out health monitoring efforts. New health norms were reinforced by health officers, residents' committee members, and workers and students themselves, as they were encouraged to monitor health behaviors of fellow workers and students. Citizens from all levels of society were supposed to be on the lookout for negative public health behaviors among their acquaintances and friends, and many acted the part.

Anti-spitting was one area for peer-on-peer monitoring. A great deal of public health materials sought to rectify this behavior. For instance, one 1953 poster uses side-by-side panels depicting a factory and a school to instruct workers and students to use spittoons. In Figure 3.3, the poster on the factory wall reads, "Be fastidious about sanitation; raise production efficiency." On the opposite panel, the blackboard instructs, "Children need to prevent TB; get the BCG vaccination" (SATA 1953–1954). Another poster (Figure 3.4) depicts children playing on the ground, presumably in a residential area, to emphasize who would be harmed by indiscriminate spitting. In the poster's image, a man carrying a book on health knows better than to spit on the ground. The red door hanging appears next to the children and reads, "Each and every household is hygienic and spotless" (SATA 1953–1954). Use of posters within the posters suggests the didactic function public health posters played in the lives of workers and students. They served as constant reminders to pay attention to health and hygiene. Public health materials reinforced basic health messages, such as hand washing or keeping streets clean. Implicit (and sometimes explicit) in the materials is an expectation that citizens would monitor the behavior of other citizens.

Persons who lived through this era, such as my interviewees, remember the constant presence of posters more than 50 years later. For instance, husband and wife, Wang Hongtie and Lu Jinling, whom I interviewed separately, remembered posters from their earliest days of school in the 1950s.[9] Wang Hongtie was born in 1951 and became a sanitation officer at a large store. His wife, Lu Jinling, was born in 1954 and was the director of a silk-spinning factory in the 1980s. These interviewees grew up with constant reminders: "Don't spit just anywhere" (不要随地吐痰). When I asked them about the Patriotic Hygiene Campaign, they recalled roles children were expected to play in environmental sanitation. My interviewees conflated the Patriotic Hygiene Campaign with Four Pest Elimination (除四害) and described the actions they took.[10] According to Lu, in the 1950s, the first problem to overcome was that of feeding the people, so the four pests endangered the people's health by increasing demand on the grain supply. She remembered participating in the campaign against sparrows as a very young child; children beat on pots and pans to frighten the sparrows so that they could not land. Her husband continued, "Students were also sent to the river to look for mosquito eggs." To eliminate rats, they used poison and two

---

9. These and all other interviewee names are pseudonyms.
10. The campaign known as Four Pest Elimination coincided with the Great Leap Forward, starting in 1958; however, pest elimination was also part of the Patriotic Hygiene Campaign following a 1952 incident of alleged US germ warfare (Rogaski 2002).

Figure 3.3: Anti-spitting poster

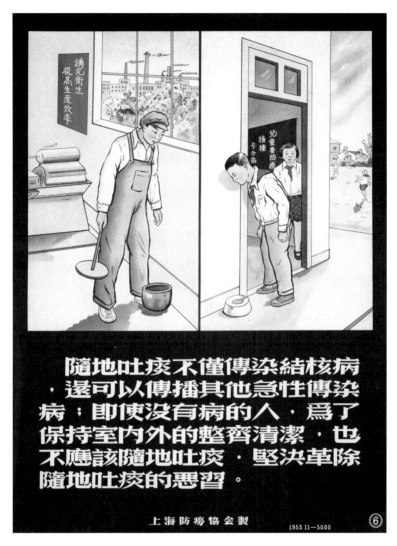

SATA 1953. The poster emphasizes, "Spitting just anywhere transmits TB and other communicable diseases." Courtesy of the United States National Library of Medicine.

Figure 3.4: Anti-spitting poster

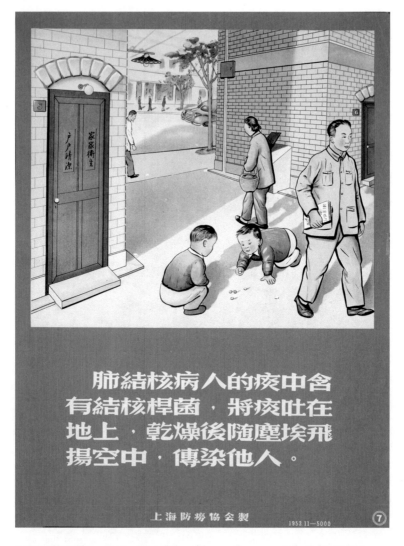

SATA 1953. This poster notes, "The phlegm of persons infected with TB contains the TB bacillus. If that phlegm is on the ground, it can be transmitted to other persons." Courtesy of the United States National Library of Medicine.

Embracing a New Scientific Health Image 93

types of traps, a box trap and a traditional baited mousetrap. Lu Jinling remembers that people were praised for turning in rats' tails. To eliminate flies, they used fly swatters and sticky/fly paper. Success in the campaign was measured by how many flies their school put in a glass jar.[11]

In some cases, children also took the health messages home to their families, potentially catalyzing a bit of reverse socialization. For example, a cartoon printed in the biweekly periodical *Combat Tuberculosis* (抗痨) in early 1958 depicts children learning about and practicing spitting into a spittoon in school. The child then brought his knowledge into the community: When the child encounters an adult spitting on the floor, he lugs a spittoon to the man's side, only to have the adult ignore the spittoon and continue to spit on the floor. The child then stands on a stool and holds the spittoon up to the man who seems surprised to have a young person correcting his behavior ("Humorous Reading" 1958). While the cartoon was meant to be funny, it also contains elements of truth: children did receive health instruction in school, and they were encouraged to share this information widely with friends and family. Although not all children would have acted on these instructions, some probably did. Reminding one's classmates and family members to spit in the spittoon was a tangible act of public health monitoring. People were given a role, and some chose to actively embrace it. In the case of children, their health awareness was only being formed, and adopting the message was part of their health socialization.

Indeed, not all sophisticated urban residents would have been willing to "get to work" (人人动手) to implement health campaigns as encouraged (SATA 1953–1954); however, use of X-ray equipment was widely documented. Mass radiography was an important part of 1950s–1970s tuberculosis control worldwide, relying on mobile X-ray units (Golub et al. 2005). China began heavily promoting mass radiography as the number of X-ray machines available for anti-TB work expanded (Wu 1947). Statistics presented at the 1956 Shanghai Municipal Anti-TB Work Representative Meeting quantify the number of group health checks being done in different types of work units between 1949 and 1955 (Table 3.2, SMA B168-1-818). These data indicate that while schools were the initial target of group health checks in 1951, workers in factories also began to be targeted over the next few years.

What sort of TB prevalence was found during these extensive health checks? Another document notes that the municipal-level tuberculosis prevention and treatment clinic, three SATA clinic outpatient departments, and Shanghai Medical College Pulmonary Department conducted 343,991 group health checks between January 1950 and December 31, 1953 (SMA B242-1-530). Of

---

11. Evidence of Four Pest Elimination has been widely cited in other works on this period. See Chang (1991) and Shapiro (2001).

Table 3.2: Number of chest X-rays by institution

	1950	1951	1952	1953	1954	1955
Factories		5,125	23,804	31,378	54,677	72,148
Schools		15,184	26,931	33,713	43,180	51,812
Government		3,477	7,296	8,694	1,193	1,293
Other		488	1,943	12,432	1,335	1,328
Total		24,274	59,974	86,217	100,385	126,581

Source: SMA B168-1-818, "1956 Shanghai Municipal Anti-TB Work Representative Meeting Documents."

the persons checked, 14,892 were found to have active disease, for a prevalence rate of 4.34 percent. Wu Shaoqing's work reported similar findings: an average prevalence rate of 5 percent for 1950–1952. Thus, in an estimated population of 5 million, the total number of TB patients might have been 250,000 (Wu 1952).

Given this high prevalence, Wu noted that it would have been ideal to do a thorough checkup of the entire population; however, in the early 1950s "manpower, material-power, and financial-power were inadequate." Wu suggested that focal points for disease monitoring efforts should be identified, so "a smaller amount of money could be spent with more efficient results" (Wu 1952: 34–35). TB prevalence was estimated to be 9 percent among industrial and commercial workers, 8 percent among public school workers, and 5 percent among university students. Based on age, TB prevalence was highest among those ages 20 to 45. Consequently, young workers and students became the target of mass radiography and group health check efforts, and mobile X-ray vehicles were sent to work units, including factories and schools.

Although the total number of individuals checked in 1955 was only half the estimated number of cases in Shanghai, the China Medical Association claims that as the decade progressed, "more than one million people were checked in an average year" in the municipality (CMA 1997). This number seems extraordinarily high; however, archival documents suggest that it may have been achievable: by the latter part of the decade, each of the four municipal clinics checked an average of 100–200 people daily (SMA B242-1-530). If each municipal clinic checked only 100 persons per day, five days per week, for 50 weeks of the year, the number of persons checked annually per clinic would reach 25,000. With four clinics, the number of persons checked could have easily reached 100,000. However, the municipal clinics were not the only facilities providing group health checks and chest X-rays. By the end of 1953, there were a total of 115 facilities using X-rays, 788 personnel who worked with X-rays (including factory and school doctors), 81 X-ray machines, and 151 TB specialists throughout the city

(SMA B242-1-530). Shanghai would have been able to reach 1 million persons per year only if each of the remaining 77 X-ray machines in city were doing an average of more than 11,000 X-rays per year, or about 45 X-rays per machine per weekday.

Shanghai had embraced a case-finding model that emphasized use of mass radiography, but not all places throughout China could do so with equal vigor. Urban areas, such as provincial capitals and other industrialized cities, had more money to invest in these efforts, but many did not begin this work as early as did Shanghai. In neighboring Jiangsu Province, the provincial capital performed chest X-rays on a mass scale, though perhaps not on as wide a scale as Shanghai. Between 1954 and 1957, Nanjing did health checks on 176,000 persons in schools, as well as industrial and mining enterprises (CMA 1997: 105). Farther from the coast, in the provincial capital of Shanxi, the Taiyuan Municipal TB Prevention and Treatment Hospital did 52,836 lung check-ups in 51 factories, mines, schools, and agencies between 1955 and 1957 (CMA 1997). Widespread use of chest X-rays allowed these cities to begin to understand TB prevalence within their boundaries, but not all cities had this sort of monitoring capacity, and rural areas certainly did not.

Where adequate personnel, facilities, and equipment existed to ensure widespread monitoring capacity, important questions remain: How did people receive these health checks? Did students and workers willingly participate? Little evidence of resistance to workplace and school health checks is found in archival documents and official sources, but there is some. For instance, SATA's 1952 work summary notes increasing prevalence among factory workers, from 5.71 percent in 1951 to 5.8 percent in 1952. SATA explained this in the following way: "Last year, not all persons participated; perhaps those who knew they were ill did not participate. This year was stricter, so persons who wanted to avoid checkups due to illness could not" (SATA 1953b). SATA's work summary does not delve into the reasons persons who knew they were ill might not want to participate; however, it is not difficult to imagine how those with little prior experience with the health system might have avoided the checkup. Perhaps these individuals were afraid of the cost treatment would entail. Perhaps they were concerned about the X-ray technology itself. Perhaps they were afraid of being fired or blocked from future employment opportunities. Likewise, given that TB had been a death sentence for many sufferers prior to the discovery and distribution of antibiotics, some persons might not have wanted to know that they had the disease (Core 2019).

To avoid workers skipping checkups, education was conducted in concert with monitoring to help allay workers' fears. SATA asked factory unions to divide workers into groups and explain how treatment would work for persons found to be infected (Song 1953). SATA posters from 1953 depicting mobile

X-ray stations emphasize "TB is easy to treat"—particularly when it is discovered early (Figure 3.5, SATA 1953–1954). As the next section describes, with widescale distribution of effective antibiotics, TB finally became easier to treat. In addition, the poster emphasizes that even healthy people should get an X-ray with the goal in mind of "early detection, early treatment." In this way, monitoring for both disease symptoms and disease progression were cast in a much less threatening light, making it more likely that workers would embrace the recommended health intervention.

Understanding the burden of infections and treating sufferers was the key to bringing high mortality and prevalence under control. In the workplace, the collection of statistics on the number of workers tested, treated, and cured was an important part of infectious disease monitoring. During the 1953–1957 First Five-Year Plan, health benchmarks encouraged participation from workers. A 1956 public health brochure, *The Work of Sanitation during the First Five-Year Plan*, by Vice Minister of Health Cui Yitian, contains a number of benchmarks to be achieved by 1957. Statistics are presented as bar graphs showing progression to the benchmarks in a manner that could be monitored by common people (Cui 1956). Similarly, a 1953 SATA poster juxtaposes the rising production rate to the falling rate of lost labor due to illness (Figure 3.6, SATA 1953–1954). The workers depicted in the poster take an active part in understanding the relationship between these variables and sharing it with their fellow workers. While requiring chest X-rays and keeping health statistics might be seen as an act of state control over the population, the idea of mutual monitoring among workers or students of the same social position and active involvement in production of statistics does not fit a top-down model. The work-unit structure facilitated both vertical and horizontal monitoring. Involving masses of workers and students and directing their attention to their own role in public health monitoring became an important part of this Communist-era project. Much of this monitoring was done in schools, factories and other workplaces where the link between health and achievement or production could be even more clearly established.

Implementing Tuberculosis Treatment

Case finding results in the reduction of active disease transmission only when the commitment to provide treatment follows, which can only be met with adequate medical personnel, facilities, and resources. As highlighted in Chapter 2, prior to the 1940s, TB treatment generally entailed rest in isolated facilities. Between 1943 and the early 1950s, discovery of effective antibiotics began to shift treatment to chemotherapy; however, until a 1956 study in Madras, India, demonstrated that TB chemotherapy worked just as well for outpatients as for hospitalized individuals, many places throughout the world continued to treat

Figure 3.5: Mobile X-ray unit

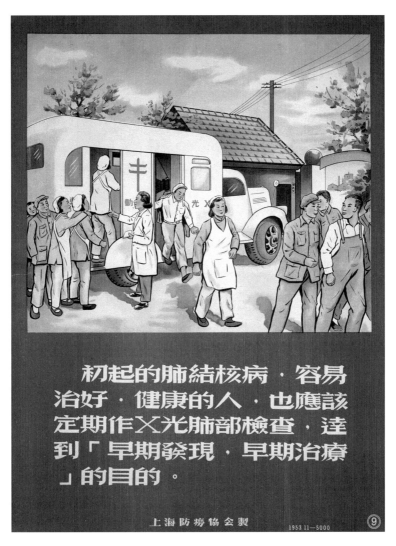

SATA 1953. The poster emphasizes, "Early stage TB is easy treat. Healthy persons should also get an X-ray to check for TB. This would reach the 'early detection, early treatment goal.'" Courtesy of the United States National Library of Medicine.

Figure 3.6: Health and production are inseparable

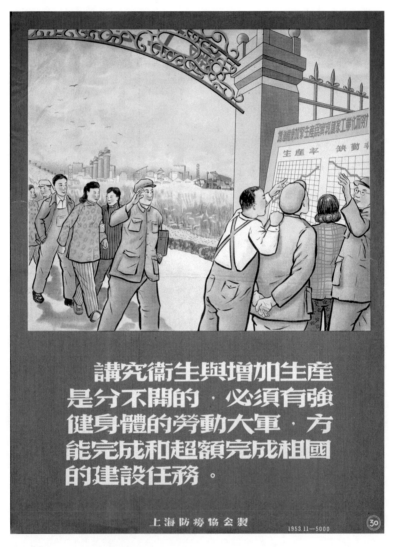

SATA 1953. The display that is the focus of the workers' attention reads, "Improve health and increase production for the purpose of realizing the country's industrialization." The graphs show rising production rate and falling loss of labor rate. Courtesy of the United States National Library of Medicine.

Embracing a New Scientific Health Image   99

TB patients in sanatoria. Moreover, as effective antibiotics were discovered, there also needed to be a means of manufacturing them and delivering these advances to the public. This section details the CCP commitment to expanding healthcare facilities and personnel, providing insurance for workers, and granting access to Western medicine and improved nutrition. Having consistent access to treatment lowered mortality rates and ultimately, incidence and prevalence rates by preventing secondary infections.

Commitment to access involved building treatment facilities throughout the nation. By the end of the First Five-Year Plan, the country's goals included increasing the number of beds in hospitals by 77 percent (to 40,000), tripling the number of beds in sanatoria and infirmaries to 55,000, and increasing the number of disease control clinics by 65.1 percent to 17,000 (Cui 1956). These goals pertained to developing facilities to treat all diseases, not just TB, and suggest that the government had ambitious plans for improving population health throughout the nation.

Given its status as the leading disease, TB received special attention in Shanghai. Prior to 1949, only 841 beds in Shanghai's hospitals were designated for TB. Wu Shaoqing estimated that 250,000 TB cases (based on a 5 percent prevalence) would need approximately 30,000 TB sick beds: "The difficulty TB patients now have in entering the hospital is that they sometimes need to wait 2–3 months for a free bed" (1952: 35). During this time, infections continued to spread. To decrease patients' wait times, the city expanded the number of beds available and imposed restrictions on which TB cases could receive hospitalization. Between 1949 and 1953, the number of designated TB beds in Shanghai more than doubled, from 841 to 2,115. Restrictions on which TB cases could receive hospitalization were used in the city's two specialized TB hospitals—the Municipal TB Hospital (with 414 beds) and SATA's First Hospital (with 160 beds)—which also helped to free up beds for patients who needed them the most (SMA B242-1-530). These facilities determined that those who needed to stay in the hospital for a short time following an operation should take priority. Hospitals could not take in severe cases and those who were unresponsive to treatment. There was also a specialized policy on limiting hospital stays. While the number of beds was still a far cry from the 30,000 Wu Shaoqing claimed were needed, the increase signaled a growing commitment to providing treatment.

Many workplaces also built "infirmaries" (疗养所) designed to treat a host of diseases, including TB. In 1954, there were 230 beds in this type of facility located throughout Shanghai, 76 percent of which were designated as TB beds. Work units with infirmaries included the Ocean Shipping Supervision Bureau (with 45 beds), Nanshi Private Treatment Hospital (with 24 beds), Hongqiao Private Treatment Hospital (with 40 beds), and Shanghai Children's Treatment Hospital (with 15 TB beds). Additionally, 19 workplaces, such as the *Liberation*

Daily (*Jiefang ribao*, 解放日报) and Xinhua Bookstore, built TB infirmaries (疗养室). Universities were one of the most comprehensive workplaces in terms of benefits provided to their members. Universities with TB infirmaries included: Caijing (with 119 beds), Tongji (with 70 beds), Shanghai Medical College (with 64 beds), East China Normal University (with 40 beds), and Jiaotong University, which increased its number of beds between 1951 and 1953 (SMA B242-1-530). Indeed, the number of beds in workplace self-built infirmaries continued to expand throughout the 1953–1957 First Five-Year Plan. In 1956, the Shanghai Central Union Workers Treatment Hospital had 600 TB beds. It would treat more than 10,000 workers in the following ten years. By 1958, the number of self-built TB beds in Shanghai's workplaces totaled 2,290 (CMA 1997).

To help meet demand for this rising number of hospital and sanatorium beds, the city also pushed to expand outpatient treatment for TB patients. In what is today Jing'an District, a number of facilities were set up, including outpatient facilities, which administered TB medication. In 1951, the Post and Telecommunications Hospital started a pulmonary outpatient department. Likewise, in 1952, the First Workers Hospital set up a pulmonary outpatient department, and a public TB outpatient department was founded in 1953 (at 885 West Nanjing Road) to provide service for 400,000 public servants (Yin 2000). Having conveniently located facilities near workplaces and residences meant people were more likely to use them. Workers and urban residents also received encouragement from their workplace leaders, health worker visits to workplaces, public health groups, and residents' committee members.

As new facilities developed, increased staffing was also needed. Nationally, the goal was a 74.3 percent increase in the number of doctors to 47,000 (including 4,000 practitioners of traditional Chinese medicine) and more than doubling the number of students enrolled in advanced training in the health professions (Cui 1956). Of course, China had a plurality of medical personnel at this time, and biomedical doctors were expected to learn some tenets of Chinese medicine. Recent historical accounts suggest that Vice Minister Cui's estimate of the number of personnel trained in biomedicine might have been an undercount. Soon (2020) estimates that almost 16,000 emergency medical personnel were trained in short-term classes between 1938 and 1946. Scheid (2002) places the number of medical personnel above 36,000 in 1949. He argues that the CCP was successful in expanding this number between 1950 and 1980, with declining emphasis on traditional medicine.

With respect to TB control, prevention nurses, whose education work was described above, worked alongside doctors. A goal of TB prevention nurses was to increase the efficiency of hospital bed usage. These nurses were sent into homes to guide severe cases who were released from hospitals because they were unresponsive to treatment (Wu 1952). The nurses provided instruction on how

Embracing a New Scientific Health Image

to isolate the TB sufferer and keep other family members safe within the home. In this way, human resources helped to compensate for the lack of physical infrastructure for treatment.

But simply providing facilities and personnel without improved commitment to covering treatment costs was not enough. In the early 1950s, the government also began to cover the cost of care through the workplace. In March 1951, the central government passed a resolution to provide health insurance for workers through individual workplaces beginning in May 1951 (SATA 1953–1954). An article in *Health News* (健康报) on January 31, 1952, lauded the advantages of this insurance in creating healthy workers (Wang Yun 1952). The article tells the story of a worker in a water bottle factory who had endured stomach pain for 10 years and was finally able to see a doctor because his work unit provided health insurance. The worker's anxious state during his illness made his head hurt. But when this worker received his union representative's assurance that medical costs would be covered, his worries disappeared. Now no doctor would turn him away because he could not pay. While this article was CCP propaganda, it was through such announcements that workers learned about the new entitlements, which were obviously a major change in their lives.

One of my respondents, born in 1928, contrasted the type of care he had received prior to 1949 with the care his factory provided when he was found to have TB in the 1950s. Four of the 10 children in his family—two brothers and two sisters—died from illnesses. His family was so poor that his mother usually used ashes from the Buddhist temple mixed with water or lotus tea as medicine. As a child, when he had a serious ailment, which turned out to be a kidney infection, a doctor wrote a prescription, but his family could not afford the medicine. Eventually, after his family appealed to the doctor regarding their financial situation, he was able to get the medicine for free. At that time, he wanted to be a doctor so that he could save people's lives. After 1949, he instead learned to fix cars and worked in a diesel factory for more than 30 years as a quality control inspector. His factory had 10,000 employees, all of whom had a card for health insurance. He stated, "If the doctor in your factory clinic had no way to help you, they would send you to a hospital." In 1957, he discovered he had TB through an examination by a mobile X-ray unit that had been deployed to his factory. He went to the hospital and then a sanatorium for one year where he took both isoniazid (INH) and a bitter decoction of Chinese medicine. With the exception of meals while he was hospitalized, his factory paid for the entire cost of treatment, something clearly unprecedented in his earlier life (Healthcare Recipient 8).

This retired worker's story seems common. Almost everyone I interviewed who lived through this era knew fellow workers, family members, or neighbors who were treated for TB. My respondent who participated in hygiene campaigns as a child, Wang Hongtie, had an aunt who suffered from TB in the 1950s, and she stayed at the hospital, where she took both Chinese medicine and isoniazid. Wang does not remember the precise length of his aunt's stay—three to four years—but he remembers going to see her on weekends. One of the things that Wang remembers was that in the hospital, TB patients had very good nutrition. While most urban residents could purchase only a small amount of rice using grain coupons, TB patients were not subject to these restrictions; instead, they ate according to their doctor's recommendations. Wang confirmed that the Communist Party did not require any money for treatment as long as you were part of a work unit. Access to free treatment, including Western medicine, and better nutrition gave TB patients much higher hopes for recovery than in the past.

Everyone I talked to over the age of 50 knows that the basic treatment regimen for TB sufferers involved taking medicines, such as streptomycin and isoniazid. The CCP emphasized making antibiotics available to workers; sometimes Chinese medicine was also recommended, often to mitigate side effects (SATA 1953–1954, M.-s. Chen 2001, Taylor 2005). China was at war when the first effective TB antibiotic, streptomycin, was discovered in 1943. Consequently, this discovery had little immediate impact in the lives of the millions of people stricken by TB. Fortunately, when isoniazid was discovered, the country was much more stable and even began producing the drug domestically at a military hospital in Shanghai in May 1952. It was then analyzed at Shanghai's First Medical College and in clinical trials in 16 hospitals (including TB Prevention and Treatment Hospitals, Zhongshan Hospital, and Huashan Hospital) from September 1952 to March 1953 (SMA B242-1-530, CMA 1997). Patient X-rays before and after intervention allowed for comparison and suggested that this domestically produced isoniazid had high effectiveness, low toxicity, and few side effects (CMA 1997). It could be produced cheaply, so in 1953, the Ministry of Health began promoting it in every city throughout the country. As the decade progressed, development of the work-unit system allowed the vast majority of urban dwellers to overcome the financial difficulty of obtaining this new medicine. Many urban dwellers without work units—such as children, retirees, and housewives—were able to rely on the work unit of a relative to provide half the cost of care, sometimes the entire cost (Providers 17 and 25).

Certainly, this model was the ideal, and it worked fairly well in China's most developed municipalities, which had greater access to resources than much of China. The model was also implemented in other provinces, but the extent of its implementation depended on the resource endowments of the location in question, including the level of training of health personnel. As an example, the *Shandong Provincial Health Gazetteer* reported that chemical treatment was not initially standardized in the 1950s, so treatment work was not widespread and the results were not ideal (*Shandong Provincial Health Gazetteer* Editorial Committee

1991: 416). If Shandong faced difficulties despite its relatively advanced economy and location in coastal China, provinces in the western hinterland surely faced even greater problems.

Conclusion

During the middle part of the twentieth century, China made great improvements in TB control. To explain advances against TB elsewhere in the world, other scholars have considered the role of environmental factors, improvement to living standards, and medical improvements, such as vaccines and antibiotics. These factors also undoubtedly contributed to the remarkable decline of the TB in China, where an effective infrastructure system for delivery of prevention, monitoring, and treatment was based in the workplace. The previous chapter argued that the GMD vision for health fell short because it did not develop an effective grassroots infrastructure for implementation. Certainly, some health programs (such as mass vaccination) that would become hallmarks of the Mao era were actually piloted during the GMD era. However, GMD-era health programming largely failed to adequately pitch the prevention message to common people, such as workers, and failed to institutionalize an effective delivery point for case finding and treatment. Consequently, care was left largely in the hands of the individual and the family. By contrast, the Communist program in the early 1950s emphasized widespread prevention programming, checkups and peer-on-peer monitoring, and supervised treatment by credentialed physicians, all delivered through the workplace.

As the CCP developed the work-unit system between 1950 and 1957, workplaces and schools became important delivery points for TB prevention, monitoring, and treatment. In the realm of prevention, the work-unit structure allowed for improved general health, delivery of inoculations, dissemination of public health materials, and public health programming designed to involve laypersons. Early Communist-era monitoring emphasized the use of mobile X-ray units and attention to public health behaviors. Widespread case finding was needed to bring epidemic TB, which had increased during the Japanese Occupation of Shanghai, under control. Workers and students were expected to be involved in the production and monitoring of health statistics and monitoring health behaviors among colleagues and friends. Some residents, including young children, enthusiastically met the new health expectations, and structures, such as sanitation teams, put in place to monitor compliance. Even if not everyone participated, the number who did impacted TB infections. Treatment in isolated facilities using Western medicine became a new possibility for many urban residents. In the 1950s, isoniazid greatly improved TB patients' chances for recovery, and the work unit helped to make medical advances available to most persons in urban areas. By 1957, most urban residents had a connection to work units. Even patients who were not employed by a work unit could receive care at facilities with support from a family member's work unit. The work-unit structure also helped to ensure compliance through its many levels of social control. Each of these developments helped to contribute to the falling TB mortality, incidence, and prevalence.

4

Shanghai's Great Leap Forward in Tuberculosis Control, 1958–1992

In November 1957, Mao visited Moscow. In response to Khrushchev's declaration that the Soviet Union's economic output would overtake that of the United States in fifteen years, Mao vowed that China would overtake England by 1972. This declaration resulted in increased agriculture and industrial targets in the PRC, which Mao thought the country could accomplish by mass mobilization and accelerated collectivization (Dikötter 2010). The Great Leap Forward (GLF) was the outcome, and Chinese from all walks of life were asked to participate in the movement. Among them, children scoured the ground for stray pieces of metal, and housewives turned in spare pots and utensils to melt down in backyard furnaces so the nation could improve its steel production (Chang 1991). Individuals would no longer need pots because communal dining was to replace private kitchens. During the summer of 1958, famine conditions appeared in many parts of the countryside, but rural areas were still expected to procure grain to feed the cities. The harvests of 1959 to 1960 were no better, resulting in tens of millions of villagers' deaths from starvation. Many statistics about industrial output during the GLF obscured the scope of the famine. Not until recently have scholars started to uncover the extent of the damage (Yang 1996; Dikötter 2010; Zhou 2013). Thus, contrary to what its name suggests, the Great Leap Forward was a devastating movement that resulted in tens of millions of deaths.

This chapter examines an area in which China, by contrast, unequivocally made great strides at this time: in the realm of TB control. An examination of TB control is particularly relevant to the period starting with the GLF because TB afflicted individuals during their prime working years and was a leading cause of missed work due to illness. Consequently, it needed to be controlled so it would not interfere with production. As noted in Chapter 3, TB was the leading cause of death in Shanghai in 1956, but Shanghai made great strides in the next few decades. By 1983, TB was only the 10th—most frequent cause of death (CMA 1997). Initially, TB prevalence rates were also extremely high, but they declined dramatically in the following decades. In 1957, prevalence was estimated at 4,200 per 100,000 residents in urban areas of Shanghai. In 1979, the TB prevalence fell 91.2 percent to 370 per 100,000, and by 1990, it dropped another 87.8 percent from 1979, to 45 per 100,000. In 1990, the published prevalence for the whole municipality, including both urban districts and rural counties, was 64 per 100,000, down 98.4 percent from 1957 (Sun 1981; CMA 1997). How did this leap forward occur?

As the nation's most industrialized city from 1949 through the 1980s, Shanghai's gross value of industrial output exceeded that of all other provinces. This industrial tradition meant that Shanghai had the organizational structure, infrastructure, and workforce to make a "leap forward" starting in 1958, which it would do by further emphasizing heavy industry. The structural transformation of industry in Shanghai actually began shortly after the 1949 Communist victory. Textiles made up more than 62 percent of Shanghai's gross value of industrial output in 1949, and heavy industry made up only 13.6 percent of GVIO that same year. In 1957, the proportions of GVIO from heavy industry and textiles were both about 36.5 percent (Howe 1971, 1981; Yan 1985). In 1958, Shanghai annexed 10 outlying counties to provide the city with the food and raw materials it needed. During the GLF, the proportion of GVIO from heavy industry swelled to over 50 percent. Following the GLF, Shanghai, like much of China, experienced economic contraction; however, heavy industry continued to dominate Shanghai's economy through the 1970s. Shanghai became the country's second-largest steel producer, as well as a leading producer of chemicals and electronics (Howe 1981). Given Shanghai's heavy industrialization, it is a good case for looking at the role of the urban workplace in TB control.

This chapter examines how work units cooperated with district-level prevention and treatment clinics to bring public health and medical advances to the public. Other recent scholarship has examined how the arrival of the 1961–1963 global cholera pandemic in Wenzhou prompted social restructuring and created systems of surveillance, ultimately consolidating state control (Fang 2021). TB was less acute and deadly than cholera, so as had been the case in the 1910s, controlling TB did not have quite the same urgency. Shanghai's concentrated battle against TB began more than 15 years before Wenzhou's battle with the cholera pandemic. As the previous chapters illustrated, Shanghai began to focus on TB as the leading infectious disease in urban areas right after the Japanese Occupation ended, and TB was an immediate focus of the new Communist government after it came to power. Urban and industrial areas emphasized the link between disease control and production at worksites starting in 1958. These sites then became the delivery point for successful TB control, which helped to consolidate state control over the citizenry.

Shanghai's Great Leap Forward in Tuberculosis Control　107

This chapter focuses largely on Yangpu and Xuhui Districts for several reasons, despite the fact that both are outliers, rather than typical districts. Yangpu presents a good case because it was home to many large factories, such as the Shanghai Bicycle Factory, Shanghai Cigarette Factory, and numerous large textile factories. Yangpu was also the home to universities including Fudan University and Tongji University, and well as the municipality's leading TB hospital. As noted in Chapter 2, this hospital had been established in 1933 as the Chengzhong Hospital and later became the Shanghai Pulmonary Hospital. Because Yangpu had many large factories, it became the model for implementing workplace-based programs. It could readily embrace the TB prevention and case-finding model recommended at the municipal level.

While Xuhui District did not have as many large factories as did Yangpu District, it did have more than 800 workplaces, including educational institutions, such as Jiaotong University, the Shanghai Medical College, and the Shanghai Library. The case is also historically interesting because the structure that became Xuhui's prevention and treatment clinic in 1958 had previously served as SATA's Shanghai Hospital, from January 1939 to June 1942. From 1944 to 1956, it served as a private hospital before being nationalized. Finally, it became the Xuhui District Tuberculosis Prevention and Treatment Clinic (徐汇区结核病防治所) in September 1958 (Mei, Zhong, and Wang 1991).[1] The example of Xuhui helps to illuminate cooperation and follow-up between different levels of the TB network in terms of case finding and treatment. The Xuhui District Prevention and Treatment Clinic was located only a few blocks away from of the Zhongshan Hospital, the tertiary-level facility that served as the teaching hospital for the Shanghai Medical College. As will be illustrated below, the Xuhui District Clinic also worked very closely with grassroots facilities on issues of staff training.

For both districts, I obtained retrospective clinic reports, issued when the clinics closed in the early 1990s. These reports contain data regarding the number of TB immunizations, screenings, and treatments implemented during the years that the clinics existed. District prevention and treatment clinic reports also provide a historical account of the clinics as workplaces, including the number of persons employed and types of benefits offered to each of them. Thus, the clinic reports serve as a record of how the clinics themselves functioned as work units, providing nutritional, health, and practical benefits to workers. For instance, the Yangpu District Clinic provided supplements for 18 types of necessities, including transportation, towels, soap, toilet paper, and feminine hygiene products (YDTPTC 1992). Likewise, the Xuhui clinic provided cloth, meat,

---

1.　In several places, I shorten "Xuhui District Tuberculosis Prevention and Treatment Clinic" to "Xuhui District Clinic"; likewise, I shorten "Yangpu District Tuberculosis Prevention and Treatment Clinic" to "Yangpu District Clinic."

108   *Tuberculosis Control and Institutional Change in Shanghai*

and grain tickets for its employees. The Xuhui clinic also raised pigs, and one interviewee confirmed that this was to provide supplemental protein to make up for the inadequate nutrition of employees, especially during the GLF (Mei et al. 1991; Provider 18).

I interviewed retired doctors who worked for or with both clinics. In the case of Xuhui, I interviewed three doctors who worked at the district clinic, as well as doctors who worked at the Zhongshan Hospital and a workplace clinic. Data gathered from these respondents figure prominently in this chapter's analysis. In the case of Yangpu, I interviewed doctors who worked both at the Municipal TB Hospital and at a large work unit within the district. Certainly, respondents took pride in their work—as well they should. Are their accounts believable, or should we view them with skepticism, given that interviews occurred 50–60 years after the events themselves? Memory can be fleeting and subject to confirmation bias, so we should approach responses skeptically. Instead of asking about specific instances, I largely asked my respondents to talk about process and trends. I jogged my respondents' memories in several ways. I brought poster images to these interviews, as well as skeptical questions about what I read in reports. Thus, while respondents were unable to talk about what happened on specific dates, they were able to describe general TB control efforts. They could talk about who was involved in BCG inoculation campaigns, describe how they cooperated with other facilities to identify cases, and verify that compliance with treatment was often a problem. Although they were eager to take pride in the change their workplaces helped to engender, they were also honest about some inefficiencies in the system. As an example, some doctors talked about how forcing busy medical professionals to attend political meetings was a waste of their time.

This chapter examines how a workplace-based tuberculosis control model allowed protocols to be implemented at a grassroots level in urban China. While China was largely excluded from international organizations, including the World Health Organization, and was increasingly isolated after the Sino-Soviet split in 1960, it is worth noting that many of the TB control protocols implemented in Shanghai were in line with the protocols being implemented at other global locations. The chapter will illustrate not only how the TB control model should have worked, but also how it did. As noted in the previous chapter, by 1957, urban residents were supposed to be members of work units. Shanghai's Great Leap Forward helped to pull many of the remaining population into the productive sector in just a few years. As the 1960s progressed, sending youth down to the countryside also helped to rectify the problem of youth unemployment and create near full employment in urban areas. However, despite efforts to push the urban population into them, not all urban residents had work units, or relatives with work units, to give them access to the workplace-based welfare system. For example, persons who retired prior to 1949 did not receive benefits

Shanghai's Great Leap Forward in Tuberculosis Control   109

through this system. Consequently, as will be described below, the TB control network also reached beyond the workplace; parts of the network also worked with neighborhood committees. Thus, while the system was designed to be largely workplace based, efforts were also made to compensate for incompleteness in that system.

Urban Health Improvements

Part of the socialist modernization project aimed at overtaking England, launched during Mao's 1957 meeting with Khrushchev, included improving hygiene knowledge and reducing lost labor due to illness. Health movements were part of a set of wider reforms, which included a 12-year plan for scientific development (Z. Wang 2015; Schmalzer 2016). As part of the movement, in 1959, the Shanghai Science and Technology Press edited a brochure called *Shanghai Hygiene: The Experience of First Entering the Work Units* on the experience of bringing general health improvements to the parts of the city. It focused on the development of mass hygiene campaigns through discussion meetings, poster exhibits, slide shows, movies, artwork, reporting meetings, and the like. The health improvements made in workplaces included a 1958 requirement for elementary school children to bring their own clean washcloth to school; this reduced incidence of trachoma by 73.6 percent. Other health interventions undertaken in the work units included ceremonial pest elimination and periodic improvements to sanitation, such as proper disposal of garbage and sewage to reduce incidence of gastrointestinal illnesses, which were particularly rampant during the summer months.

Targeting TB in the factory

TB was particularly important to the health improvement agenda because it was one of the leading illnesses that contributed to lost labor; consequently, it called for social reform. At the beginning of the 1950s, TB was framed as a disease of capitalist exploitation—poor living and working conditions made workers susceptible. By this logic, industrial campaigns with lofty output targets, such as the GLF, had the potential to prompt a resurgence of TB by encouraging workers to neglect their health in favor of production. Instead, the health rhetoric of the GLF continued to emphasize the need to eliminate TB so it would not interfere with production. The 1959 brochure, *Shanghai Hygiene: The Experience of First Entering the Work Units*, also talks about the number of TB sufferers at the Shanghai Smelting Plant. A high number of respiratory disease sufferers might be expected given that smoke and other lung irritants were present in the factory. Among the suggested health improvements at this factory were to keep

Figure 4.1: Tuberculosis incidence for Yangpu District

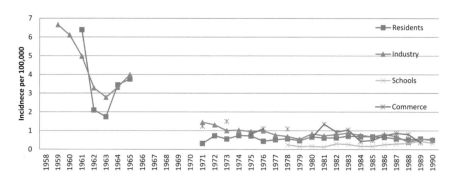

Source: 1992 *Chronicle of the Yangpu District Prevention and Treatment Clinic.*

TB patients' bowls and chopsticks separate from those of healthy people and to finally eliminate the perpetual nuisance of indiscriminate spitting. While separate eating utensils is more relevant to gastrointestinal ailments, the brochure demonstrates that both hygiene and TB were concerns in industrial workplaces.

The Shanghai Smelting Plant was just one of many factories with TB problems. In heavily industrialized Yangpu District, TB was the reason behind much of the lost labor due to illness. In the early 1960s, there was some fluctuation in TB incidence, as efforts were made to reduce lost labor. According to a 1960 archival document, of 161,649 workers checked in 104 factories, 6,324 (or 3.91 percent) had TB. While a slightly higher number actually had high blood pressure, TB was most severe with respect to work absences. Consequently, bringing down incidence was part of the prevention and treatment plan (YPA 47-13-62). The actual rate of lost labor from TB appears to have been higher than the incidence rate, based on the 1960 checkups, very likely because some patients with TB discovered in previous years continued to recuperate. By the end of 1961, TB absences were somewhat reduced. According to an archival document from November 4, 1961, 1,468 persons had been diagnosed with TB in 125 factories and two hospitals since June 1960. The rate of lost labor from TB for the third quarter of 1961 was 4.4 percent, approximately half of what it had been one year prior (YPA 47-13-70).[2]

Fluctuations in the data suggest the challenges of bringing a highly infectious disease under control. These fluctuations make the data seem more

---

2. According to this document (YPA 47-13-70), the rate of lost labor from TB was 8.6 percent in the third quarter of 1960.

believable than if they formed a neat and continuous downward trend. There is really no way to confirm their veracity, but looking long term, a downward trend is evident. According to the 1992 *Chronicle of the Yangpu District Tuberculosis Prevention and Treatment Clinic*, incidence among district residents was 6.39 per 100,000 in 1961. Incidence then fell in 1961 and 1963, before rising in 1964 and 1965. Among industrial workers, incidence dropped consistently between 1959 and 1963, only to rise in 1964 and 1965. Part of this 1964–1965 increase might have been residual health problems from the Great Leap Forward. Unfortunately, data are not available for the early Cultural Revolution (1966–1970), but when data started to be gathered again in the 1970s, a downward trend was evident, with some year-to-year fluctuation (Figure 4.1). These sorts of improvements came about both as a result of general disease prevention campaigns, as well as health-care access improvements offered through the work-unit system.

Structure of the urban healthcare system

By 1958, a three-tiered system of urban health care was fully in place in Shanghai. As noted in the previous chapter, starting in the early 1950s, workplaces provided medical insurance to employees, meaning that they agreed to cover the costs for all medical treatments associated with illness. All workers with a work unit had a designated hospital they were supposed to visit when injured or ill. Where they went depended on the organizational position of their work unit. In general, municipal-level hospitals served mostly state-owned enterprise employees and dependents, often following referral from workplace clinics. District-level facilities served collective enterprise employees and their dependents. Workers from smaller workshop enterprises went to neighborhood hospitals and clinics. At these facilities, incurred costs were covered or reimbursed through one of two systems. The labor insurance system (LIS) covered workers in factories, mines, and the transportation system, as well as 50 percent of costs for these workers' dependents. The government insurance system (GIS) covered government workers—for example, employees of schools, hospitals, banks, shops, restaurants, and government offices (Tang and Meng 2004).

Many large workplaces had their own onsite clinic or hospital. For most ailments, workers simply went to their own clinic or designated hospitals. Workers could then receive a referral to higher-level facilities depending on the severity of the illness. Statistics in archival documents suggest that areas with a high concentration of factories also had numerous workplace clinics and hospitals. For instance, in 1960, Yangpu District had 290 factories with 245,000 workers. In 1960, 92 percent of the 151 factories with more than 300 workers had health stations: 119 (78.8 percent) had established permanent health stations, and 20 had mobile stations (YPA 47-13-62). Factories in the district also committed to expanding medical personnel in the workplace. Between 1957 and 1960, factory medical service workers increased 37.6 percent (from 921 to 1267): doctors increased from 155 to 261, and nurses from 329 to 485 (YPA 47-13-70). Some workplace facilities had numerous doctors and saw large numbers of patients. As an example, the Yangpu Cotton Factory Hospital saw 70,435 outpatients during the second quarter of 1961 (YPA 47-13-70). While these data might not be completely accurate, the intention was certainly to provide health services to workers.

In practice, the three-tiered system ensured that some workers had better access to health facilities than others. While the 1960 report from Yangpu emphasized that 92 percent of factories with more than 300 workers had a clinic or mobile clinic, it said little about the 139 factories with fewer than 300 workers. It is possible that some of the health needs of workers in smaller factories were also well served, but I found evidence of heterogeneity of services between levels of the municipal health system. Naturally, urban residents wanted to receive care for themselves and their sick family members in top-level facilities, even if their workplace affiliation did not entitle them to do so. In a 2011 interview, a retired doctor from a university hospital noted that many patients sought care at a tertiary-level hospital and falsely claimed affiliation with the university. These opportunistic individuals knew that the tertiary hospital was the municipal-level facility designated to treat students, faculty, and staff, with conditions that the university hospital was unable to treat. Their behavior forced the university to revise its payment policy in the early 1960s. Instead of paying the hospital directly for its affiliates' clinical care, the university required its affiliates to pay at the time services were rendered and seek reimbursement (Provider 25).

TB Control at the Height of the Work-Unit System

In the realm of TB control, there were also three levels of facilities, and an effective TB control network was created to overcome the heterogeneity of the system. Each level had specific tasks with respect to record keeping and reporting, staff training, and TB control interventions. The municipal-level prevention and treatment clinic kept records on disease reporting throughout the municipality, set policy, and helped to steer disease prevention and treatment activities in lower-level facilities. District-level facilities played a crucial role coordinating with facilities above and below them. District prevention and treatment clinics sent medical staff to municipal hospitals for the purpose of continuing education. Likewise, municipal hospitals sent medical interns to district prevention and treatment clinics to do rotations. Similarly, medical staff from district prevention and treatment clinics went to grassroots facilities to train factory and other workplace doctors, and workplace doctors went to district clinics for certain types of training. In general, personnel from district clinics coordinated with staff at grassroots facilities to bring prevention activities, case finding, and treatment to the population. Medical personnel from district prevention and treatment clinics worked with school doctors to administer BCG shots and boosters in schools and to workplaces to take chest X-rays, identify TB sufferers based on X-ray slides, and oversee treatment (Mei et al. 1991; Provider 18). I describe some of these efforts in more detail below.

The three-tiered infrastructure of urban TB control, which reached maturity around the time of the GLF, was actually initiated during the First Five-Year Plan. In some places, construction of the crucial middle tier of the system in fact commenced at the beginning of the First Five-Year Plan;[3] however, most of this mid-level infrastructure did not develop until the end of the First Five-Year Plan. In 1957, Luwan and another urban (sub)district built prevention and treatment clinics. In 1958, eleven more urban districts (including Yangpu, Xuhui, Changning, Putuo, Huangpu, Zhabei, and Hongkou), four of Shanghai's rural counties (Shanghai, Jiading, Baoshan, and Chuansha), and the Shanghai Railroad Bureau built facilities (CMA 1997). While the number of district prevention and treatment clinics would change over the years as some districts (or subdistricts) merged with others,[4] something that did not change was the crucial role they played in coordinating with workplace doctors to bring health to the masses.

The following subsections examine TB preventive programming, case finding, and treatment efforts, most of which were designed to reach members of the population through their work units. As noted above, despite its exclusion from the WHO, many of the protocols that China implemented were in line with the international health protocols being recommended worldwide. They included the BCG vaccine for infants and children, health education to raise awareness of disease symptoms and encourage reporting, case finding through mass radiography, and treatment using antibiotics. Only with respect to treatment did China deviate from international health protocols: doctors in Shanghai readily embraced and promoted antibiotics as part of the cure for TB, but their recommendations regarding rest in designated facilities were stricter than those in some other global locations. As mentioned in the previous chapter, in 1956, isolation was no longer recommended for TB sufferers receiving chemical treatment; however, this section will illustrate that Shanghai continued to build and maintain isolation facilities in the 1960s and sometimes even into the 1980s.

---

3. Songjiang County built the rural equivalent of a district-level clinic in 1953.
4. For instance, the Xincheng and Jiangning District Clinics merged to form the Jing'an District Clinic in 1960 (Yin 2000). Likewise, Yulin and Wusong District Clinics combined with the Yangpu District Clinic as the Yangpu District incorporated more land (YDPTC 1992).

114   *Tuberculosis Control and Institutional Change in Shanghai*

Shanghai's deviation from global protocols may have stemmed from limited space to isolate TB sufferers in their homes.

Strengthening TB prevention efforts

As demonstrated in the previous chapter, the Chinese Ministry of Health promoted widescale BCG inoculations of infants and children throughout the nation in the early 1950s. By the time of the GLF, BCG inoculations had become systematized among infants and children. Testing to assess reactivity to the bacillus—and thus whether booster shots were needed—also became a standard intervention. In a 1958 article, the Shanghai Health Bureau enumerated the goal of follow-up testing: All of Shanghai's 1 million children under the age of seven were to be tested in the following six months. Children were given skin tests, and those who were nonreactive received a BCG booster (Shanghai Health Bureau Prevention Office 1958). Archival documents suggest that the bureau was successful in this bid. On May 18, 1959, the municipal-level tuberculosis prevention and treatment clinic reported that in 1958, 14 district and county clinics in Shanghai examined 1,041,217 children under age 15, followed by 530,831 shots. The clinics also vaccinated 183,365 newborn infants (SMA B242-1-1176). While these data are impossible to verify, providing BCG was among the important work of district (and county) clinics. High numbers of inoculations continued throughout the GLF. Between 1958 and 1960, approximately 2,390,328 inoculations were given to children, and the number of infants inoculated reached 80 percent throughout the municipality (SMA B242-1-1510; Core 2014).

    The district prevention and treatment clinics helped achieve high BCG rates by developing programs to target newborns in maternity wards and children in schools. Both programs involved cooperation between district clinics and other work units. Inoculation of newborns depended on cooperation with hospital maternity wards, where infants received BCG. These hospitals reported BCG inoculation numbers to the district TB prevention and treatment clinic at set times. Every year, the district clinics' BCG nurses went to the maternity hospitals and wards to inspect infant vaccination records. In Xuhui District, four hospitals immunized newborns in the early 1960s: the International Peace Women and Children's Health Protection Hospital, Rijun Hospital, Zhongshan Hospital, and the Shanghai Electricity Hospital (Mei et al. 1991). Where a pregnant woman went to give birth was determined by her work unit, or her husband's work unit. The Xuhui District Clinic also kept tabs on babies of district residents who were not born in any of these hospitals, which was important for persons who were not affiliated with work units. BCG nurses were sent to residences to inoculate these infants. In this way, district clinics sought to reach persons without work units who might be missed by the system.

The 1991 *Chronicle of Xuhui District Tuberculosis Prevention and Treatment Clinic* also describes the clinic's strategy for providing BCG booster shots to children who were previously immunized as infants. Each year before the boosters were done, the district clinic would hold a training session for all elementary and middle school health teachers in the district. At these annual meetings, personnel from the district clinic and from schools discussed public health education and BCG coverage, and also planned the inoculation schedule. School personnel were vital to this process. Health teachers took responsibility for organization, mobilization, and consolidating the list of children to receive boosters, as well as keeping their family heads informed. Prior to 1981, children received boosters at the ages of one and four, as well as in the first year of elementary school, first year of middle school, and second year of high school (Mei et al. 1991).[5] Before administering boosters, the clinic used tuberculin skin tests and gave chest X-rays to children with a strong positive reaction.

The Xuhui District Clinic oversaw the administration of as many as 30,000 shots annually before the Cultural Revolution, with more than a fifth given to newborns. In 1964, maternity wards gave 5,289 initial doses, and schools gave 22,491 boosters. District personnel claim that inoculation coverage rates for newborns were consistently maintained at 99 percent (Providers 18 and 20). However, because inoculation data are not available from the Cultural Revolution, this claim is hard to substantiate. Certainly, the administration of BCG to newborns was already institutionalized as a health practice prior to the Cultural Revolution and women still gave birth during these years, but in some areas of Shanghai, backsliding may have occurred with respect to BCG administration.[6] Throughout China, children could not enroll in school unless they had received doses of BCG, and they could not remain enrolled without having scheduled checkups and any necessary boosters. In my interviews, doctors credit this policy with helping to lower TB prevalence throughout the city and nation (Provider 32).

In other districts, BCG immunization planning took place in a similar manner. Recommendations regarding the booster schedule changed somewhat over the years, but district clinics implemented the policies set at the municipal level. Each year, in Yangpu District, teachers and street-level doctors received training before administering the vaccinations in schools. Between 1958 and 1990, the Yangpu District Clinic held 20 BCG training sessions (YDTPTC 1992). During these same years, maternity wards and schools provided 1,770,242

---

5. In 1981, the number of times BCG was to be administered to children changed: at birth, during the first year of elementary school, and the first year of middle school. Consequently, the total number of BCG boosters being administered fell.

6. Chapter 5 provides evidence suggesting that BCG coverage rates dropped in one of Shanghai's rural counties during the Cultural Revolution.

inoculations and reported them to the Yangpu District Clinic. This number seems insignificant given that in 1958 alone, more than 1 million children were tested throughout Shanghai, but the numbers from multiple clinics across Shanghai's districts would have added up.

Naturally, Shanghai was not the only city to prioritize BCG during the GLF. Making BCG available was a national policy. At a TB control conference held in Shanghai in June 1963, doctors from around the nation determined that in urban areas, BCG inoculation rates had reached more than 90 percent for newborn infants (Xinhua 1963). Inoculation rates would continue to rise and would remain high through the following decades. Certainly, as Mary Brazelton points out in *Mass Immunization*, it is possible that statistics were inflated. Perhaps doctors at the 1963 conference were afraid to admit challenges to their efforts because they did not want their locality to look bad; however, TB fell dramatically, and increasing use of BCG was part of the explanation.

Another area for primary prevention was health education. As described in previous chapters, some of this education aimed to change health behaviors, such as indiscriminate spitting in public places and other behaviors believed to spread disease. Health campaigns also sought to make the population aware of disease symptoms to encourage self-reporting to treatment facilities. This enhanced case finding was led by district prevention and treatment clinics and delivered in work units. With the aim of interrupting the disease transmission cycle and bringing down the rate of lost labor due to illness, the number of preventive programs increased dramatically during the GLF. Because Yangpu had many large factories, the Yangpu District Clinic put effort into factory education, but factories were not the only target. After the clinic's founding in 1958, TB prevention knowledge and programming in the form of pictures, slideshows, and reporting on blackboards in cafeterias and near entrance gates was shown to approximately 9,500 persons in more than 100 factories, schools, and residences (YDTPTC 1992). Thus, the attempts at health socialization using visual imagery described in the previous chapter became institutionalized.

In 1959, the Yangpu District Clinic continued to lead the "leap forward" through its educational programming. It made 14 TB prevention movies available to 12 large factories, where 11,200 spectators viewed them. While this was only a fraction of Yangpu's workers, health messages reached workers in other ways as well. Factories held exhibits featuring 1,855 posters, such as those discussed in Chapter 3. Before annual health checkups, work units also did a media blitz; they used broadcasts, blackboard reporting, propaganda posters, and lectures to make workers aware of the importance of getting checked, both for their own health and for the sake of production. The Yangpu District Clinic selected workers to write about their experience with TB control, resulting in 12 brochures, which the district clinic disseminated in 1959. The district clinic also arranged 372 lectures for TB patients at their work units with the goal of preventing spread of the disease and ensuring compliance to treatment regimens (YDTPTC 1992).

Certainly, TB prevention programming was widespread, but was it effective? Were workers able to balance participation in health programs with production? According to one of my respondents, who worked in a district prevention and treatment clinic, since there were so many preventive programs being held in the factories, workers were not required to attend this programming (Provider 18). This respondent said that workers needed to work in order to meet production targets. While workers might not have been able to attend all programs, the anti-TB messages were all around them. Each year in the early 1960s, the Yangpu District Clinic supported some sort of TB prevention propaganda. For example, a factory and work unit TB prevention class was held each year to train medical service workers. In addition to doctors, factories had health teams whose members were picked from among workers to help promote programming and encourage adoption of recommended healthy behaviors. By 1960, Yangpu factories had chosen more than 6,300 workers to join health teams (YPA 47-13-62). That year 218 factories used blackboards posted in cafeterias and near the factory gates for TB prevention, and 172 factories used announcements. About 47,000 persons attended 1,265 slide shows, and 23,500 people also watched one or more of 38 anti-TB films screened in work units. Archival documents do not specify the location of these slide shows or movies, but factories, schools, the Hudong Workers' Cultural Palace, and even some residential compounds assisted with this programming.

Factories and other workplaces were certainly not the only locales where preventive programming was provided. The district clinic's propaganda vehicle also went to the streets, reaching 155,000 district residents. Likewise, workers' palaces were community centers with exhibit spaces and auditoriums used for films, performances, and lectures. Given the large number of workers in Yangpu District, the Hudong Workers' Cultural Palace had many programs, including health-related ones. The Yangpu District Tuberculosis Prevention and Treatment Clinic often cooperated with the Hudong Palace in health programming and encouraged workers to get involved themselves. For instance, the auditorium of the Hudong Workers' Cultural Palace showed TB prevention slides to 155,000 people (YDTPTC 1992). In 1961, a small publisher also started a collection of art and culture on TB control done by district workers at the palace. Encouragement of worker involvement was not just limited to print media. The Yangpu District Clinic created a prize and encouraged workers to create their own theater performances focused on TB control. In 1961, 12 factories and work units performed 14 shows. Three outstanding shows received prizes (YDTPTC 1992). This type of programming not only encouraged workers to internalize the anti-TB message;

it also allowed them to improve upon the message in ways that resonated with workers. Thus, the district clinic capitalized on workers' free labor to improve its message.

Similar programs were held at the street level. While there is no way to assess the reception of street-level programming, one of my interviewees who worked at the Xuhui District Tuberculosis Prevention and Treatment Clinic claimed that residents were even more welcoming of lectures than were workers. Their clinic worked closely with street-level hospitals and neighborhood committees to do this sort of outreach when they found numerous TB patients in one area. The purpose of this work was to increase self-reporting in places with high incidence rates (Provider 18). The need for outreach to residential areas implies that the reach of the work-unit system was never as pervasive as municipal disease control authorities might have liked.

Many preventive education programs ceased during the early years of the Cultural Revolution, 1966–1968; however, by the early 1970s, some of the district prevention and treatment clinics had started to recover prevention work. During the 1970s, the Xuhui District Clinic held meetings to discuss the experience of TB prevention in factories throughout the district. For example, on the afternoon of October 4, 1973, the Shanghai Sixth Fermentation Factory held an anti-TB meeting where several other factories all presented their respective work units' anti-TB development situation and results (Mei et al. 1991). These events suggest that while there was a temporary hiatus, workplaces, such as factories, continued to cooperate with one another and share experiences in disease prevention as soon as the situation was more stable.

Case finding and treatment

In addition to primary prevention programs, active case finding, which started in the early 1950s, was further systematized during the GLF. Each of the district (and county) clinics had X-ray equipment, but the actual number screened per district varied from year to year. I discussed active case finding with retired doctors who considered ACF to be the clinic's most important work (Providers 18 and 20). These findings illustrate close cooperation between district prevention and treatment clinics and workplace clinics during collection and monitoring of chest X-ray slides and throughout treatment of any TB patients discovered through ACF.

The general trend that emerges from the data is of a push to find those with active TB during the Great Leap Forward and early 1960s. In the Xuhui District alone, 140,000 individuals were screened in 1964, but the number of screenings declined after this because of a number of factors (Core 2019), among them the turbulence of the Cultural Revolution, when many doctors were criticized.

Shanghai's Great Leap Forward in Tuberculosis Control

Following the Cultural Revolution, there was a slight uptick in the number of screenings in 1979, only to resume the downward trend in the 1980s. Perhaps most important was the fact that by the end of the 1960s, they were not finding as many TB cases through X-rays, so they stopped doing them as frequently. After the initial GLF push, the number of persons discovered with active disease as a proportion of the total screened began to decline. Many large units that systematized the practice of annual screenings would continue to hold them throughout the 1980s, but some switched to biennial screenings, and others began to implement passive case finding (Provider 20). Xuhui's shift away from active case finding reflects wider global shift to passive case finding during this period as well (Golub et al. 2005).

Providers 18 and 20 both described the process of going into factories in Xuhui District, taking chest X-rays, and identifying potential TB sufferers during the clinic's early years. Provider 20 said that they could do as many as 200–300 checkups a day (or about 25–40 per hour) in workplaces during the 1960s. During an interview, I expressed skepticism about whether quality could be maintained when they were doing such volume; each worker would have had only two minutes with the provider. The retired doctor laughed and said the only thing these checkups included was X-rays. They did not measure workers' weight or do any other type of health tests. They also did not analyze the X-rays or make diagnoses until a later date. They simply sent two vehicles to take chest X-rays. Unlike public health programming, these checkups were generally mandatory for workers. Provider 18 concurred regarding what "checkups" entailed: chest X-rays were the only thing included. Many could be done, and they were a big money maker for the district prevention and treatment clinics. Work units paid a 4–5 RMB fee per checkup for all workers as part of their insurance. There were more than 800 workplaces, including over 100 factories in Xuhui District. Since the clinic did 100,000 X-rays per year, the district clinic made a good deal of money from these checkups (Provider 18).

Most of the district's 710,000 residents of working age were employees of its 800 work units, but what happened to persons who were not formally employed? Sometimes residents were able to get chest X-rays at other locales. Provider 18 stated that the Xuhui District Clinic seldom used the X-ray vehicle at the street or neighborhood level, but when it did, it provided free services. People who did not have work units simply did not have the same sort of systematic inclusion in annual or biennial active case finding as did employees in factories and govern-ment offices. Provider 18, who liked to practice English with me on occasion, switched to English to emphasize this point: "Common residents couldn't enjoy annual checks," but the district clinic for which he worked tried to make check-ups more widely available.

After they had collected all of the X-rays, diagnosis was the next step. Doctors from the Zhongshan Hospital trained district clinic doctors in reading chest X-rays prior to the Cultural Revolution. Workplace and district clinic doctors then worked together to view the small X-ray slides to identify potential TB sufferers. Provider 18 said that it was easy to identify potential TB sufferers because their lungs had lots of cavities and looked like the painted face of a Chinese opera character (*dahualian* 大花脸). When the clinic was founded, there were many of these. Later, there were very few (Core 2014). After two to three doctors looked at the slides, suspected persons were asked to come to the clinic to have a big film taken. The clinic also asked for a sputum test, which their laboratory staff processed.

In Yangpu District, workplace doctors also collaborated with the district clinic on the issue of diagnosis. According to the district clinic report, diagnosis took place one day every week. Every two weeks, the district scientific association also held a meeting for the specialized study of TB diagnosis. Sometimes the meetings were also open to doctors from grassroots facilities. At the Yangpu District Clinic, for example, 800 workplace doctors participated in X-ray-card-reading sessions during the years the Yangpu clinic was in existence (YDTPTC 1992). The work of identifying cases was an important step in stopping disease spread.

After diagnosis, treatment is the next step in TB control. As mentioned in the previous chapter, based on the results of the 1956 Madras study, which found patients are no longer infectious approximately two weeks into a course of antibiotics, TB sanatoriums began to close worldwide (Toman 1979). Despite the emphasis on biomedicine, Shanghai continued to isolate TB patients because many were unable to self-isolate for the first two weeks of treatment in their crowded urban residences. The Great Leap Forward saw a continued push for TB patients to receive treatment in isolated facilities to minimize the danger of infecting their friends and family. As noted in the previous chapter, large factories and workplaces set up their own infirmaries for TB patients starting in the 1950s, and this continued through the GLF. Eventually, when the number of TB cases throughout Shanghai municipality declined, the number of designated TB beds in the city also started to decline.

Workplaces continued to build and maintain treatment beds during this time. In 1958, the number of sick beds in Shanghai work-unit infirmaries totaled 2,290, and this number expanded in the next few years (CMA 1997). In Yangpu District, seven large factories established 197 TB beds by 1959. In five of the factories, self-built TB infirmaries were relatively short lived, corresponding roughly to the years of the GLF. The largest was the Twelfth National Cotton Factory, which had 35 beds from 1957 to 1959. The smallest was at an auxiliary power plant, which had 12 beds from 1957 to 1963. Among the other factories,

Shanghai's Great Leap Forward in Tuberculosis Control 121

the Ninth and Nineteenth Cotton Factories, also had self-built treatment rooms for a decade or more (YDTPTC 1992).

Yangpu District also had a number of beds in both TB-specific and general hospitals. In addition to the Shanghai Pulmonary Hospital, which had 605 beds, and the Yangpu District Prevention and Treatment Clinic, three additional hospitals in the district had designated TB beds: the Yangpu Central Hospital, the Xinhua Central Hospital, and the Second Textile Factory. These wards were set up during the GLF. The Second Textile Factory ward remained open until the 1980s, and the Xinhua Hospital TB facility remained open until 1990 (YDTPTC 1992). The ongoing presence of TB beds at the Second Textile Factory and Xinhua Hospital into the 1980s suggests that isolation in Shanghai continued for decades after much of the world moved away from the model of isolating TB sufferers.

Not all districts had as many designated TB beds. In Xuhui, the district clinic had some TB beds, and some work units within the district such as Jiaotong University had infirmaries, but the district clinic's main emphasis was on outpatient treatment using antibiotics. In Xuhui, persons found to have TB were registered at the district prevention and treatment clinic. Registration cards were used to ensure treatment compliance. When completing the cards, medical personnel asked questions such as, "What medicine did the patient take? When did the patient need to do reexamination?" (Provider 18). When disease registration and reporting began at the time of the clinic's founding, doctors were responsible for the registration cards. District clinic doctors worked closely with doctors in workplace and neighborhood facilities to monitor treatment progress. In 1972, responsibility for registration cards in Xuhui District shifted to nurses.

Even with the multiple levels of surveillance, compliance with chemical treatment regimens was always a problem among patients because the treatment was lengthy and involved a combination of antibiotics, many of which caused uncomfortable side effects. When doctors were in charge of registration cards, patients had to report to the district clinic once every two weeks throughout their lengthy treatment. While workplaces excused these workers, reporting to the clinic was still inconvenient, so patient management was always an issue. Clinic staff would often have to seek out TB patients who missed appointments (Provider 20). Doctors at workplace and neighborhood facilities also tried to ensure that patients came to their appointments. A doctor who worked at a university hospital reported that work units were responsible for making sure patients from their workplace properly followed treatment. Specialized municipal-level clinics decided the treatment course—that is, the combination and length of antibiotic treatment. Doctors at municipal-level clinics shared this information with the district clinics, who in turn told workplace doctors how to treat patients. Doctors at the district clinic each had books of registration cards, and workplace doctors, such as my respondent from a university, went to the district clinic for training (Provider 21). Provider 20 believed that the Xuhui District Clinic had a good relationship with work units in the district. His impression was that the doctors at factories and schools oversaw treatment very well. He lauded these close working relationships as one of the important factors that had contributed to the sharp declines in TB in the 1950s and 1960s. While it is possible that this doctor misremembered (or misrepresented) much about the process, I have little doubt that patient compliance was a tricky issue, requiring cooperation from multiple levels of Shanghai's TB control network.

Keeping close tabs on patient registration cards was also important and challenging work in Yangpu District, particularly after the number of beds in workplace treatment rooms began to decline. According to the 1992 *Chronicle of the Yangpu District Tuberculosis Prevention and Treatment Clinic*, when there were so many patients in the 1960s, the reexamination situation was taken very seriously because declining TB might reduce workplace illnesses. But by the end of the 1960s, some compliance problems emerged. In the Longjiang Street neighborhood in 1969, an astounding 22.7 percent of 673 cases stopped taking their medicine on their own, and 39.2 percent had their treatment canceled for some other reason, which left only 38.1 percent who complied with treatment. This signaled to the Yangpu District Clinic that it needed to provide better oversight of treatment in both workplaces and neighborhoods. For more than 10 years thereafter, the Yangpu District Clinic paid attention to this, collaborating with the Shanghai Number One Iron and Steel Plant, Hudong Boat Factory, China Boat Factory, and Meizhou and Pudong Street Hospitals to correct the approach to treatment.

In June 1977, the Yangpu District Clinic strengthened its management of patients undergoing treatment. One doctor and two nurses took responsibility for 134 cases. They kept records, held card-reading meetings, and conducted three large patients' meetings to do educational work. They also sought to do reexaminations on time and according to the patient supervision plan. Within nine months, the rate of transformation of sputum smear tests (from positive to negative) was 96 percent, and the rate of people returning to work was 76 percent (YDTPTC 1992). Thus, even as China began to turn toward market socialism, TB treatment remained a priority.

How was the treatment of patients who were discovered through visits to residences, rather than visits to workplaces, managed? The Xuhui District Clinic also worked with street-level hospitals and neighborhood committees and sent nurses to families. When the Xuihui District Clinic was founded, the only street-level hospital with a pulmonary department was the Industrial and Agricultural Hospital. In 1960 and 1961, Caobei Neighborhood Hospital and Xinle Neighborhood Hospital founded pulmonary departments. In 1972 and 1975, the Xu and Yongjia Neighborhood Hospitals also founded pulmonary departments. These neighborhood hospitals were responsible for TB prevention, checkups, and treatment on their own streets and on behalf of the Xuhui District Clinic. They gave relevant statistics to the Xuhui District Clinic each year. At the street level, independent health protection stations were still under the direct supervision of the district TB prevention and treatment clinic (Mei et al. 1991).

In the 1980s, nurses from district clinics were particularly important in reaching patients at the street level, who were not otherwise served in workplace clinics. These public health nurses took responsibility for treatment cards and would go to patient homes to make sure they were taking medicine for the full course. Nurses also schooled the patients in basic infection prevention: "Don't cough, don't spit, sterilize chopsticks, etc." (Provider 18). House call cards were completed by nurses at the time of their visits. The majority of the Xuhui District Clinic's nurses did house calls. Each nurse had a neighborhood for which they were responsible. The nurse went there once every two weeks, which was more successful than requiring workers to come to the clinic had been in the 1960s. The clinic would keep disease registration cards until it was totally cured, usually two to three years. They required patients come back for follow-up appointment, but only a few did (Provider 18).

The example of nurses from the Xuhui District clinic going to neighborhoods demonstrates that some district facilities reached out to urban residents who did not have a work unit. Public health nurses monitored the treatment of these individuals—keeping track of their patient management card and visiting them at home every two weeks for two to three years until their illness was totally cured. Unfortunately, try as they might, clinic staff could not enforce treatment follow-up as well in neighborhoods as the factory and other workplace doctors could. Workplace doctors, in contrast, could continue to require all employees to get chest X-rays on an annual basis to make sure their TB did not recur, whereas the street-level nurses did not have a comparable infrastructure to enforce follow-up checks.

The Xuhui District Clinic also provided free antibiotics to those who did not have a work unit and were in a precarious financial situation. The clinic began providing this service to long-term residence permit (*hukou*) holders under financial hardship in August 1959. Free and reduced-price treatment relied upon proof of a patient's financial hardship, with verification from the neighborhood committee. Patients could then enjoy care from area nurses. When the clinic first began implementing free and reduced-price treatment, there were four types: by one-third, one-half, two-thirds, and full price. If the patient experienced a change to their financial or medical situation during treatment, area nurses would adjust the level of reduced price the patient received accordingly. Provider 18 noted, "Free TB care in the late 1950s was a stark departure from the time of the Private Shanghai Hospital, when patients who could not pay couldn't enter the hospital. At that time, doctors could set up private practices in the hospital and make lots of money."

Unfortunately, free patient care was not the norm throughout Shanghai. The Yangpu District Clinic did not begin providing free treatment to those under financial hardship until 1980. Most of the rest of the district clinics did not begin providing free treatment until 1983. In some cases, TB sufferers with financial hardships were able to get free treatment at a municipal-level facility. I discovered evidence of this in my interviews with a former director of the municipal-level prevention and treatment clinic. This retired doctor still received New Year's visits from a patient to whom he had provided free treatment decades earlier. From my interviews, I was not able to ascertain how widespread provision of free treatment was throughout the municipality before 1983 (Provider 17). My interviewees who retired from the Xuhui District Clinic claim that they were the only district to provide free TB treatment. Thus, many TB sufferers in other districts might have been missed.

Regardless of inequalities of access, bringing infectious cases into treatment resulted in reduced TB prevalence in both Yangpu and Xuhui. In Yangpu, factory prevalence rates started out higher than the rates for district residents and schools. Owing to the types of interventions outlined above, prevalence in factories declined to a level approximating those of general residents in 1974. Starting in 1979, factory rates were slightly lower than general resident rates (YDTPTC 1992). These reductions in factory prevalence rates probably reflect a number of factors, including better case finding and management during treatment. In Xuhui District, a similar drop in prevalence occurred, particularly among state-owned factories, financial institutions, and government offices. Between 1959 and 1990, prevalence rates for every level of enterprise in Xuhui District dropped greatly: 96.3 percent in factories, 96.5 percent in finance and trade companies, 94.8 percent in government organizations, and 90.5 percent in collective enterprises. As a result of this success, the clinic began to focus on other respiratory diseases in addition to TB. In September 1988, the clinic changed its name to the Xuhui District Tuberculosis and Lung Tumor Prevention and Treatment Clinic. The new name reflected Shanghai's changing disease burden and the shifting priorities of health resources. As infectious diseases declined and the population lived longer, chronic diseases became more prevalent. Consequently, resources once expended toward infectious disease control were shifting to combat chronic conditions. While TB remained in the clinic's name, it was no longer the sole focus of attention.

Other district TB clinics also began to shift their focus away from TB in the 1980s and 1990s. In 1987, the Zhabei District Clinic added specialized outpatient departments for lung cancer, acute bronchitis, and other respiratory infections, and it increased the number of personnel dedicated to these ailments. While this clinic had only 8 personnel (including seven technical medical personnel) when it was founded in 1958, in 1993, it had a larger and more well qualified staff, with 40 employees, including 32 medical technical personnel (Fan 1998). In some ways this shift reflects a wider shift in global health, as an epidemiological transition occurred in middle- and lower-middle-income countries, where infectious diseases had once been the primary causes of death (Chen and Chen 2014; D. Zhang 2014; Burns and Liu 2017; Liu and Krumholz 2017).

Conclusion

Certainly, not all socialist experiments were successful. Indeed, the Great Leap Forward was disastrous, but with respect to tuberculosis control, China had something to prove, and it did. TB was one of the diseases responsible for lost labor due to illness. At the beginning of the Great Leap Forward, the Chinese nation became fixated on production, so halting anything that interfered with it was a priority. Consequently, social restructuring was needed to control infectious disease and the WUS became the primary delivery point for making public health and medical advances available. TB prevention programs began to be run in factories and other work units throughout Shanghai, including both primary and secondary prevention, which aimed to interrupt the disease transmission cycle by making sure infectious patients received treatment. This identification of TB patients ranked among the most important work of district prevention and treatment clinics. Clinics worked closely with workplace doctors to identify persons with affected lungs. As fewer patients with deeply affected lungs began to be discovered, the number of annual chest X-rays declined. Once patients were discovered, workplace doctors, street-level doctors, and public health nurses from district prevention and treatment clinics enforced compliance with treatment regimens. While factory workers had access to frequent screenings and consistent care, this was not true of all residents of Shanghai; however, disease control facilities aimed to reach many of those without work units.

My empirical research findings show that general health and TB indicators improved greatly in the 1960s–1980s. Life expectancy rose dramatically over these two decades in both urban districts and the countryside. According to World Bank data, life expectancy rose from 44 in 1960 to 67 in 1980, and it kept rising beyond this (World Bank n.d.; Wang 2004; Chen and Chen 2014; Zhang 2014). Mortality and prevalence from tuberculosis also fell dramatically. In many ways we might view Shanghai's 1958–1992 TB control program, particularly the way Xuhui and Yangpu Districts executed it, as a model for all of China. Because Shanghai was already so heavily industrialized in 1958, the municipality could capitalize upon the many factories for health planning. Moreover, during the Great Leap Forward, even more of the city's residents were pulled into the city's work units—a phenomenon which also happened elsewhere in China. Shanghai's TB control network relied on hospital maternity wards and schools to carry out BCG inoculations. Persons who remained outside of work units sometimes relied on coverage from a family member. Shanghai's neighborhood committees also allowed propaganda teams and X-ray vehicles to reach some individuals who remained at home, and did not have a workplace.

Many of the disease control interventions highlighted in this chapter would continue until the 1990s in Shanghai, but not all Chinese cities were as industrialized. Consequently, work unit coverage might not have been as complete. Moreover, the majority of Chinese citizens lived in the countryside, which had a system entirely separate from the urban work-unit system. In the following chapter, we turn to disease control in Shanghai's rural counties.

5

Building and Maintaining the Tuberculosis Control Network in Shanghai's Rural Counties, 1950s–1990s

The previous chapters have argued that despite its imperfections, urban Shanghai's TB control network, which made medical advances available through work units, was a model for other Chinese provinces and municipalities to emulate. The health system in Shanghai's rural counties was a likewise imperfect model. In fact, in the 1970s, foreign delegates who came to Shanghai on "carefully choreographed" visits even upheld China's rural health system as a model for other countries to emulate (V. W. Sidel and R. Sidel 1974, 1982; Wei, Wilkes, and Bloom 1997; Brazelton 2019b; Zhou 2020: 264). The barefoot doctor program, in particular, was a low-cost intervention that could be scaled up very quickly to allow rural residents to receive basic first aid and preventive health services. Barefoot doctors worked in clinics supported by rural production brigades, which, like urban work units, helped to reach the population at the grassroots level. However, as in urban areas, health-care provision among Shanghai's rural counties was uneven. This chapter examines the creation and evolution of the health-care system in Shanghai's rural areas and the ways this system was used for TB control.

Because tuberculosis was largely a disease of crowded urban environments, it has not received much attention in the historical literature examining health improvements in rural areas. In the 1950s, TB in Shanghai's rural counties was not as prevalent as in urban districts, but it still was a serious problem, and in some counties it received attention from rural medical professionals. When the first epidemiological study of TB in Shanghai's rural counties was done in 1957, prevalence was estimated to be 45 percent lower than in urban areas.[1] From the 1950s through the 1970s, TB prevalence fell dramatically in both urban and rural areas of Shanghai. In 1979, it was estimated to be 350 per 100,000 in both areas.

---

1. In 1957, prevalence was 4,200 per 100,000 in urban Shanghai and 2,340 in the rural counties (CMA 1997).

In the 1980s, TB prevalence in rural areas began to exceed the rates in urban areas. Indeed, prevalence in Shanghai's rural areas continued to decline; however, the decline was not as pronounced in urban areas. By 1985, TB prevalence in Shanghai's urban districts was more than 20 percent lower than in the rural counties. The gap between rural and urban Shanghai would continue to widen: by 1990, prevalence in Shanghai's rural areas was 89 per 100,000, nearly double the 45 per 100,000 in urban areas (CMA 1997). The trend of rural areas outpacing urban areas was not just a trend in Shanghai. In fact, TB prevalence in rural areas, where the healthcare system is not well developed, has been driving some nationwide trends in recent decades, particularly as rural residents have migrated to urban areas (Shen et al. 2012).

The trend of rural counties driving tuberculosis nationwide has been exacerbated by disinvestment in the rural health-care system. In the 1980s, in many Chinese counties, the rural health-care system largely collapsed when the communes that financed it were dismantled (Blumenthal and Hsiao 2005). In many places former brigade-level clinics closed, but in a few other places the rural health-care system transformed. For instance, Xiaoping Fang demonstrates that in Zhejiang the number of barefoot doctors declined, but the remaining rural health practitioners were better credentialed. According to Fang, the number of village clinics in Zhejiang, especially near Hangzhou, remained anomalously high: the percentage of villages with a clinic nationally fell below 10 percent in 1983, but in Zhejiang it remained above 70 percent in 1984–1988, and near 90 percent in Hangzhou's rural areas (2012: 171–75). Likewise, this chapter examines continued investment in the health-care system and infrastructure in several of Shanghai's rural counties, which have always had an advantage over most of rural China, because of their close proximity to the economic hub. Starting in the late 1970s, Shanghai's rural counties became the site of rapid industrial development. This chapter demonstrates that when industry took off in the rural districts of Shanghai, along with other rural districts in China's coastal regions in the 1980s and 1990s, Shanghai's advantages with respect to rural healthcare became more pronounced. I focus largely on Shanghai (now Minhang) and Songjiang Counties but will also introduce data from Shanghai's other rural counties, including Fengxian, Jiading, and Jinshan. By 2000, all but one of Shanghai's former rural counties were incorporated as urban districts and were covered by the same municipal insurance as the urban districts.

Fundamental Institutional Change: Rural Collectivization and Its Implications for Health

Collectivization of agriculture began at the same time that urban industries were collectivized between 1950 and 1957. The earliest steps toward land reform came in the year immediately following the Communist victory. A land reform law adopted in June 1950 called for the redistribution of five major properties: draft animals, farm implements, houses, furniture, and land (Huang 1990). During this process, peasants were assigned to categories based on their property holdings and whether they hired labor or were hired as laborers. Landlord was the worst category; their property was seized and given to the poor peasants. Collectivization then came about through three additional steps during the 1950s, which Philip Huang describes in his work on Huayangqiao Village in Songjiang County. In 1952, mutual aid teams were set up to oversee resource pooling. Starting in 1954 with "early-stage" collectivization, production was done in a group, and yield was distributed according to household land and labor contributions. In 1956 Shanghai's rural counties achieved a "higher-stage" of collectivization, and distribution became based upon household labor contribution. During the 1958–1961 Great Leap Forward, collectivization reached completion; at the time, agricultural areas were organized into communes. The size of Shanghai's communes varied considerably, but generally communes had 10,000 to 30,000 persons.[2] Communes, in turn, were divided into production brigades. Brigades also varied in size, but generally one administrative village of 2,000 to 5,000 persons comprised a production brigade (New and New 1975).

Along with these new institutions came norms regarding what they were expected to provide for their members. After the production brigades were created, they became the key, systemic locale for reaching the population in health programming, much as work units served as grassroots implementation points in urban areas. Rural counties throughout China developed a three-tiered health-care system. The most advanced tier was the county level. County-level facilities often had a number of specialized departments responsible for tasks such as infectious disease control (including TB prevention and treatment clinics), family planning, and mental health, as well as a central general hospital. Counties were the administrative equivalent of urban districts, and the rural health system had two administrative layers below the county. One step below were the commune hospitals. In the 1980s, the communes became townships, and the former commune hospitals became township (镇 or 乡) hospitals. At the grassroots (村) level of the three-tiered structure were very simple production brigade clinics.

China made an initial foray into developing health clinics in people's communes during the Great Leap Forward. For example, in the communes around what are now Chedun Town and Sheshan Town in Songjiang District, village health clinics were built in 1957 (Zhao 2011a; Liu and Yu 2012). Similarly, in

---

2. Pickowicz (1971) estimates that Shanghai's communes had an average population between 25,000 and 30,000.

the communes in what are now Xinqiao Town and Xiaokushan Town, village health stations were set up in 1958 (Q. Liu 2011; Zhao 2011b). The existence of a few clinics in the 1950s does not signal a developed rural health-care system. Rather, it suggests that some areas with means invested in ad hoc clinics that early. In fact, Songjiang's GLF "boom" was very short lived. The county's GVIO increased from 67 million RMB in 1959, to 95 million in 1960 and 100 million in 1961, only to drop to 60 million in 1962 (Whiting 2001: 43). With economic retrenchment following the GLF, efforts to build and staff brigade clinics faltered in many areas of China (Fang 2012).

The GLF deeply affected China's rural residents and caused the state to reevaluate its approach to rural health. The great famine led to widespread malnutrition and tens of millions of deaths in the Chinese countryside. In the mid-1960s, with the recovery from the post-GLF collapse, Mao again realigned the nation's attention toward health improvements in rural areas. On June 26, 1965, he gave a speech that became known as the "June 26th Directive." Mao's words, "Put emphasis of health work on the countryside," became a guiding principle for the next several years (*China Anti-Tuberculosis Journal* editor 1965). Development of the three-tiered cooperative medical system arose from this new emphasis on rural health provision.

The CMS had a number of advantages, including cost efficiency. Because the brigade financed it, cost control was a goal. Peasants were required to pay a small portion of their income before they could receive benefits through the CMS. This fee was often equivalent to about 1 percent of a peasant's annual income, and this amount was matched by a contribution from the production brigade (V. H. Li 1975). Costs were kept down primarily through the type of medical services that were provided and the referral path. At the brigade level, medical services were limited to mostly preventive medicine, which is more cost effective than curative therapies. When curative therapies were needed and brigade clinics were unable to treat a given ailment, they would refer the case up to a commune or county hospital. Higher-level health facilities also provided regular technical assistance and supervision to brigade clinics. Thus, with respect to the referral path and technical assistance from above, the brigade clinic resembled the work-unit clinics in urban areas, which received help from district clinics.

Brigade clinics were staffed by the famous barefoot doctors (BFDs), peasant paraprofessionals who worked part time as doctors and continued to labor part time in the fields. The term "barefoot doctor" was not coined until 1968, but wealthy rural counties, such as many in Shanghai, already had health workers years before the term came into use (Pickowicz 1971; Fang 2012). Because Shanghai was China's largest and most industrialized city, it was in a much better position than most Chinese cities to provide medical training and equipment to its rural perimeter. Even before the CMS was formally established, by June 1960,

Building and Maintaining the Tuberculosis Control Network 131

there were 3,900 medical paraprofessionals in the 2,500 production brigades surrounding Shanghai. In 1968, *Red Flag* reported that its surrounding counties had 4,500 barefoot doctors. By the end of 1969, the Xinhua News Agency reported that the number of barefoot doctors in Shanghai's rural counties was 6,000, or 2.4 per production brigade (Pickowicz 1971). It is likely that some of these statistics were inflated to make the Communist health project look good during the Cultural Revolution; however, Shanghai's rural counties came to expect to have some medical personnel in the late 1960s.

The number of barefoot doctors and the brigade clinics they served continued to expand throughout the 1970s. According to a report by the Shanghai Health Bureau's revolutionary committee on June 26, 1974, Shanghai's rural counties had 2,780 brigades and 8,666 barefoot doctors (SMA B123-8-1055-22). In 1976, the same committee reported that Shanghai's rural counties had 9,634 barefoot doctors and 100 percent of its 2890 rural production brigades had implemented the CMS (Table 5.1). These figures were almost certainly inflated. Even if almost all of Shanghai's brigades made some sort of health provision, variation certainly existed between personnel training and what clinics were able to provide. In fact, as will be described below, my respondents who were sent to the countryside to provide care to rural areas acknowledged that this unevenness helped to determine where they went (Provider 20).

Not all of the approximately 70,000 people's communes throughout China had comparable health personnel and services; however, another advantage of the CMS was how quickly it could be scaled up. Between 1965 and 1980, China

Table 5.1: Grassroots brigade implementation of the Cooperative Medical System, 1976

County	Number of clinics	Number of BFDs
Shanghai	243	821
Jiading	260	794
Baoshan	204	707
Chuansha	332	1,062
Nanhui	350	1,220
Fengxian	291	1,023
Songjiang	245	820
Jinshan	211	890
Qingpu	326	940
Chongming	428	1,357
Total	**2,890**	**9,634**

Source: SMA B242-3-754-132.

trained approximately 1.8 million barefoot doctors throughout the countryside (Lucas 1980). One of the reasons this program could be scaled up so quickly was that the training they received was brief: generally three to six months, but training courses could be as short as 35 days (Hsu 1974). Scholars have pointed out that this model was not ideal—inexperienced barefoot doctors were likely to make errors—but the tasks they undertook on a daily basis did not require an advanced skill set (Hsu 1974; V. H. Li 1975). They treated basic illnesses and injuries and practiced preventive medicine—that is, immunizations, waste disposal, and maintaining clean water supplies (Young 1984). Ideally, barefoot doctors would receive additional training to upgrade their skills throughout their service, but this did not always happen. Barefoot doctors were assisted by health aids and midwives, whom they managed and trained. In 1980, there were an estimated 4 million heath aids and midwives throughout China (Lucas 1980).

In addition to being cost effective and rapidly scalable, the barefoot-doctor program had the advantage of being embedded in the communities it served. BFDs received authority from and were accountable to members of their brigades. They were often recruited or nominated based on their willingness to serve (or their political reliability), rather than any innate ability or educational background. For their efforts, they were remunerated by the production brigade in work points, just as other peasants engaged in productive labor. As a result of the program's structure, barriers between elite medical providers and their patients were also lowered. Moreover, because barefoot doctors were also peasants who toiled alongside other peasants in the field, they understood who was ill and what diseases were likely to appear at various seasons (M.-s. Chen 2001). They could better advocate for their patients at training sessions held at the commune and county level.

Owing to the scale of the system, under the CMS, health-care access ceased to be a privilege in rural China. By 1980, the system covered 90 percent of China's rural population (Liu et al. 1995; S. Wang 2004). Rural production brigades invested in the system both financially and emotionally. One scholar concerned with the development of primary health service in developing countries wrote that the CMS was the "institutionalization of people's participation in decisions which affect and improve their own healthcare" (Rifkin 1978: 34). Ideally, the system empowered peasants with the knowledge and means to protect their own health.

The CMS has been widely credited with bringing about a dramatic reduction in infectious diseases (Horn 1971; V. W. Sidel and R. Sidel 1974, 1982; R. Sidel and V. W. Sidel 1977; Henderson and Cohen 1984; S. Wang 2004; Fang 2012). However, this system also had a number of limitations. First among these was unevenness of training among barefoot doctors. Second, there were disparities of care among the types of services that rural production brigades could offer. Wealthier production brigades could afford to pay for more services. An additional limitation was that in some cases, peasants demanded more expensive medicine or treatment than was merited by their medical condition (Hsu 1974). When this happened rural production brigades would ask peasants to increase the amount they paid for service.

Recent scholarship has amplified the negative assessment on the barefoot-doctor program. For instance, Zhou Xun's 2020 monograph, *The People's Health*, investigates several problems associated with it. Among them, Zhou highlights how the program failed to incentivize ongoing medical education, especially for female BFDs. Zhou also asserts that BFDs' promotion of contraception and medicalized birth was out of step with peasants' prioritization of big families and home births. Perhaps most alarming, Zhou's evidence suggests that the distribution of antibiotics by poorly trained BFDs exacerbated the problem of drug resistance, including for TB (Core 2022). Indeed, Zhou's critique about overprescribing echoes that of other scholars about "inappropriate and excessive use of drugs" and injections at the village level (Wei et al. 1997: 37).

Overuse of drugs and increasing drug resistance are certainly alarming concerns; however, this chapter will demonstrate that the rural medical system had some success in engendering improvements to TB mortality and prevalence. The CMS structure facilitated making medical advances—such as using X-rays for case finding and antibiotics in treatment—available in rural areas. In this way, the chapter builds upon Xiaoping Fang's finding that one success of the barefoot doctor program derived from the efficacy of Western medicine. Of course, implementation of some medical advances in rural Shanghai largely occurred more than a decade later than, and less consistently than in urban areas.[3] After introducing general improvements to medical infrastructure and health in Shanghai's rural counties, the next section investigates the TB programs being implemented, primarily in Shanghai County.

Using the CMS for TB Control in Rural Shanghai

Shanghai County's cooperative medical system

Shanghai County was the closest rural county to Shanghai's urban core, sitting immediately south of the central urban district. This county shared a border with Xuhui, the prosperous district described in the previous chapter. Industrial production became increasingly important in rural Shanghai County during the Mao era. In 1967, industry already accounted for 40.8 percent of total county

---

3. While BCG campaigns in some rural areas of Shanghai occurred in the 1950s, widespread active case finding was not widely done until the 1970s.

income, and by 1980, it accounted for 65.4 percent; however, in 1980, approximately 80 percent of this county's 561,427 residents were peasants (Ye et al. 1982). In 1992, the county was renamed Minhang and was incorporated as an urban district. In 2010, the gross value of industrial output for this district was higher than for all but one of Shanghai's other districts.[4]

In 1980, the approximately 80 percent of the residents who were peasant farmers were covered under the CMS, but this coverage was somewhat uneven. In 1980, Shanghai County had 18 communes, ranging in size from 12,708 to 41,371 members, with an average of 27,264. The communes, in turn, comprised 238 production brigades. All of the 238 brigades in the county had BFDs; there were a total of 751, with an average of 42 BFDs per commune and 3–4 per production brigade (Gong and Chao 1982). The number and type of health facilities, including hospital beds per capita and number of per capita health workers, varied between communes in Shanghai County. For example, Hongqiao Commune's population was more than twice as large as that of Qiyi Commune, yet Qiyi Commune Hospital had 82 beds, and Hongqiao Commune Hospital had only 25.[5] Given its large population, Hongqiao also had a relatively high ratio of population per BFD. Hongqiao had 511 residents per BFD, and Qiyi had 442 (Gong and Chao 1982). Despite these discrepancies, all communes in Shanghai County endeavored to make health services available, including member access of higher-level facilities, as necessary. Statistics on the patient composition at the county hospital reflected the fact that peasants generally went there only if they were referred. Of inpatients at the county hospital around 1980, 57 percent were peasants who had been referred to the facility from brigade or commune clinics (Ye et al. 1982). At the county hospital, only 13 percent of outpatients were peasants because many ailments could be treated in the brigade clinics. County hospitals were often located in rural towns, where many residents had another classification of resident permit, such as industrial. Approximately 9 percent of patients who sought care from BFDs were referred to commune or county hospitals.

This snapshot of rural health services in Shanghai County is not necessarily typical of rural health service in China, but it was fairly typical of Shanghai. As another example, in 1971, the Hongqiao Commune of Chuansha County had 200 medical and health personnel for a population of 27,000. This commune had 15 production brigades, each of which had an average of 14 health workers, including two barefoot doctors. This commune's population to barefoot doctor ratio

---

4. In 2009, the GVIO for Pudong District (formerly Chuansha County) was highest, at 698.2 billion RMB, and the GVIO for Minhang District was 332.3 billion RMB (*Shanghai Statistical Yearbook 2010*).

5. Mid-1980 population for Hongqiao was 35,606 and for Qiyi was 16,286 (Ye et al. 1982).

(850) suggests an even more dire situation than at Shanghai County's Hongqiao Commune, but the barefoot doctors in Chuansha County were assisted by additional health aids (Pickowicz 1971). Moreover, because the Shanghai County statistics came from 1980 and the Hongqiao statistics from 1971, Shanghai County had an additional decade to train barefoot doctors.

Until the three levels of the rural health-care system could be developed, rural counties relied partially on mobile teams of medical personnel from urban areas. These teams made visits (巡回) to rural counties, providing training to rural health personnel on issues such as immunization and disease identification. The following section illustrates several examples.

Urban providers and the development of the rural healthcare system

In the years immediately after the founding of Shanghai's urban TB prevention and treatment clinics in the late 1950s, urban district-level facilities and hospitals sent mobile teams of doctors and nurses to the countryside to train health personnel and provide health services. For instance, the Xuhui District Clinic sent 28 doctors and nurses to make 18 visits into Shanghai's countryside between 1958 and 1978. The Xuhui clinic's attention to the countryside began right after its 1958 founding, when a nurse was sent to Chongming County for a year, but an even more concerted effort—16 of the clinic's 18 trips—was made to bring TB control to the countryside following Mao's June 26, 1965, directive (Mei et al. 1991). This district prevention and treatment clinic's rural service missions included three to Guizhou Province and two to Yunnan; however, its remaining 13 mobile medical teams went to Shanghai's rural counties, including 4 to neighboring Shanghai County.

The Xuhui District Clinic chose to prioritize Shanghai County, both because of the county's location and the holes in its rural health provision. In terms of location, Shanghai County was the closest rural county to Xuihui (Provider 18).[6] Within Shanghai County, the Xuhui clinic chose the communes to visit based on their need for health personnel. The urban medical teams went to four of the five communes in Shanghai County, which had the highest population-to-BFD ratio in 1980.[7] The importance of the Xuhui District Clinic's visits to neighboring Shanghai County is evident from a number of factors, including timing and duration of these missions, number of staff, and staff qualifications. In terms of

---

6. Provider 18 visited Shanghai County from September 1967 to March 1968. This provider also visited Songjiang County in January to March 1972 and Guizhou from July 1976 to May 1977.
7. The Xuhui Clinic made visits to Beiqiao, Minlong, Xinzhuang, and Jiwang (Mei et al. 1991), which were four of the only five communes in the county that still had a ratio greater than 500 in 1980. Hongqiao was the other county that ranked in the top five among communes with the highest population-to-BFD ratio (Gong and Chao 1982).

timing, the clinic targeted Shanghai County right at the beginning of the Cultural Revolution, and three of the four visits lasted for a year or more. Only 5 of the 18 mobile medical visits from the Xuhui clinic lasted so long. Indeed, size and compositions of the medical teams are additional factors suggesting prioritization of the visits to Shanghai County. While 7 of the 18 teams from the Xuhui District Clinic involved only a single medical provider, the three largest missions of personnel went to Shanghai County. Each of these visits included at least one doctor trained in Western medicine and three nurses. Moreover, each of these visits involved experienced doctors and nurses, two of whom had already been to the countryside in 1966 (Mei et al. 1991).

The duties that urban health personnel fulfilled when they were in the countryside included helping to train rural health personnel to execute the same sorts of TB education programs that were done in the cities. While two areas of Shanghai County had made an initial foray into vaccination in 1951, starting in 1959, urban teams helped to systematize immunizations of infants and children under 15 (Lü 1990; Mei et al. 1991). Personnel from the Xuhui District Clinic provided further training in BCG administration to barefoot doctors and other rural health personnel during their 1966–1970 visits. By the late 1970s, there were specially trained inoculation teams in the countryside (Provider 17).

Shanghai County was not the only one of the municipality's surrounding counties to receive medical missions focused on TB control. The Yangpu District Tuberculosis Prevention and Treatment Clinic also sent personnel to Shanghai's rural counties. While most of the Xuhui clinic's missions included more than one staff member, Yangpu often sent a single provider. Yangpu especially prioritized Chongming Island and Nanhui County. Twenty-seven Yangpu District Clinic personnel went to the countryside for a year or more, and three went to the countryside twice. All but 3 of these 30 mobile medical visits were to rural counties within Shanghai municipality. Nineteen of the personnel sent to the countryside from the Yangpu District Clinic spent at least a year on Shanghai's Chongming Island, and six spent at least a year in Nanhui County. Of the three personnel who did two rounds, one went to Chongming and Nanhui, one to Jiading County and Nanhui, and one to Chuansha County and to Anhui Province (YDPTC 1992). This rural-urban interaction was precisely what Mao envisioned in the June 26 Directive.

In addition to the services provided by district-level clinics, municipal-level hospitals also sometimes provided health-care to the countryside. A doctor from the pulmonary teaching and research organization at Zhongshan Hospital, the hospital affiliated with Shanghai Medical College, went to the countryside in the spring of 1965. Dr. Cui worked in the Gaoqiao and Baijia Production Brigades of the Zhongnian People's Commune in Jinshan County, Shanghai's southwestern-most rural county, which borders Zhejiang Province. Dr. Cui conducted interviews with 1,310 persons from 730 households over the course of five months. He discovered low TB prevalence among his interviewees; however, he also found a tendency to ignore early disease symptoms. Of the 11 TB patients he interviewed, most had lung cavities and waited until their disease reached an advanced stage to seek medical help (Cui 1966). Dr. Cui wanted to see improved prevention, early detection, and supervised use of antibiotics, but these suggestions could only be acted upon once the CMS was in place.

Mobile medical teams from urban areas provided a way to improve medical provision in rural areas, which did not have the resources to provide specialized care. As a final example, 13 urban hygiene work teams made visits to Jinshan County's 15 communes between 1965 and 1972, where they had 1,660 interactions with patients. The urban teams included several specialists; notable among them were internal medicine specialists, a radiologist, a urologist, and a pharmacist (*Jinshan County Health Gazetteer* editors 1994: 201). This sort of attention to the countryside was given to various locations throughout China, but implementation in most places was likely not as strong as in Shanghai, where trained medical professionals in the urban core outnumbered those in other provinces.

In the months following Mao's June 26 Directive, medical journals, such as the *China Anti-Tuberculosis Journal*, focused on bringing health to the countryside. Ten articles on rural health and tuberculosis control in the countryside appeared from late 1965 until the journal was discontinued with the 1966 onset of the Cultural Revolution, including two emphasizing general improvements to health in the countryside and eight articles focusing more specifically on TB control. The TB control articles include a directive from the PRC Ministry of Health and the National Anti-Tuberculosis Association to every province, autonomous region, and municipality on "strengthening anti-TB work in the countryside" (*China Anti-Tuberculosis Journal* 1965). Six articles were included under a banner with Mao's famous June 26 Directive, "Put emphasis of health work on the countryside," in one issue of the *China Anti-Tuberculosis Journal*. The articles focused on specific programs being implemented in rural locations throughout China and how to create the new norm of "serve the people" (为人服务). Thus, while implementation varied across China's vast countryside—with most provinces unable to provide the quality of services offered in Shanghai—certainly the intent was the same.

Using the rural health system to facilitate TB control

Some TB control efforts were made in rural Shanghai in the early 1950s, but not nearly as many as in urban areas. For instance, some counties began efforts in immunization and isolation. In the early 1950s, Jinshan County began BCG inoculations (*Jinshan County Health Gazetteer* editors 1994), and Shanghai

County implemented some BCG inoculations in Longhua and Xinjing (Lü 1990). In 1952, Shanghai County also built a 160-bed workers sanatorium (Lü 1990: 44). It was originally intended for model laborers, but in 1954 it became a chronic disease hospital, and in 1956 it became a TB hospital. A few county TB prevention and treatment clinics were also established in the 1950s, at the same time as those in the urban districts. In fact, Songjiang County established the very first county-level clinic in 1953, years before most urban districts did. Baoshan, Chuansha, Jiading, and Shanghai Counties also established clinics in 1958 (CMA 1997). However, other counties did not develop prevention and treatment clinics until after the Cultural Revolution. For instance, Nanhui set up a county clinic in 1976, Fengxian and Jinshan in 1978, and Qingpu in 1979, but this did not mean that no TB interventions had previously occurred in these areas (Fengxian County Health Bureau *Health Gazetteer* Writing Group 1985; *Nanhui Health Gazetteer* Writing Leadership Team 1987; *Qingpu Health Gazetteer* Compilation Committee 1989; *Jinshan County Health Gazetteer* editors 1994).[8] Rather, it signaled that there was not the systematic attention to intervention at the county level as there would be after the Cultural Revolution. Regardless of the date of their founding, the county-level clinics played a similar role to that of the district clinics, their administrative equivalent in urban areas.

Shanghai County has among the best-documented rural health interventions, but records also contain a few questionable claims. For instance, one retrospective source asserted that BCG rates in Shanghai County were already over 90 percent in 1958, which would have been even higher than in urban areas at the same time; however, the same source claimed that in the early 1970s, BCG rates in the county were nowhere near this level. BCG rates increased from under 20 percent in 1974 to 42 percent in 1976, to over 99 percent in 1978 (Lü 1990: 84). If BCG rates had been higher in the late 1950s or early 1960s, the 1970s data suggest that TB control in rural areas suffered setbacks during the Cultural Revolution.

Data on TB control between 1965 and 1972 are only fragmentary, and then TB control began to recover. As part of this recovery, in 1973–1975, counties began to implement surveys to better understand the disease situation. Among them, three brigades and a hospital in Fengxian County worked with the municipal-level TB prevention and treatment clinic to implement a TB prevalence

---

8. As example of TB interventions before the county clinics were established, in the 1950s Qingpu County investigated workers in Zhujiajiao Town. The survey found high prevalence (20 percent), and as a follow up measure, Zhujiajiao People's Hospital undertook childhood BCG immunizations and worked with the Zhongshan Hospital to set up pulmonary outpatient and inpatient departments starting in 1958 (*Qingpu Health Gazetteer* Compilation Committee 1989). Likewise, Fengxian People's Hospital also worked with maternity clinics to administer BCG starting in 1962 (Fengxian County Health Bureau *Health Gazetteer* Writing Group 1985).

investigation in 1973 (Fengxian County Health Bureau *Health Gazetteer* Writing Group 1985). Jinshan and Shanghai Counties also implemented mass screenings in 1974–1975 (Lü 1990; *Jinshan County Health Gazetteer* editors 1994). During Shanghai County's mass screening, all individuals 15 years and younger were given skin tests, and all individuals 50 and older were given chest X-rays. Those between the ages of 15 and 50 were given X-rays if they were found to have a history of tuberculosis symptoms, such as a chronic cough. Persons with a close contact who had TB also received X-rays. After the 1975 mass screening, case finding was generally done through passive means. Annual X-rays were given only to those at risk of contracting lung disease—for example, workers in factories, family members of TB patients, and TB hospital staff—as well as those likely to put others at risk if they contracted active TB, such as food handlers, teachers, and childcare personnel (Han and Yang 1982).

When TB cases were discovered in rural areas, what sort of treatment did they receive? In Shanghai County, patients interacted with health professionals at least every two weeks during their monitored treatment regimen. Barefoot doctors and medical personnel from the commune hospital visited patients with active disease at home every two weeks to ensure compliance with drug therapy regimens. On the first visit of the month, the BFD would bring a one-month supply of medication; on the second visit, the BFD counted the number of pills the patient had left. Medical personnel from county hospitals also made monthly visits. In part, as a result of these interventions, TB prevalence and mortality in Shanghai County declined: prevalence fell 77 percent, and mortality fell 69 percent between 1961 and 1980 (Han and Yang 1982: 48). As in the urban areas, numerous factors figure into falling mortality and prevalence, including preventive programming, early diagnosis, and treatment compliance, as well as more distal factors, such as adequate nutrition.

Other rural counties also used the three tiers of the CMS to facilitate TB control. As mentioned above, Songjiang County began to set up its anti-TB network in 1953. In July 1960, the county hospital pulmonary department created six TB infirmaries, which adopted a combination of Chinese and Western medicine to treat more than 400 cases in Chengdong Commune, Silian Yexing Brigade, Yangjing Brigade, and Yutang Brigade. After two years, five of the infirmaries closed, but Sijing's endured until 1971 (Y. Zhang 1989).[9] Given that the brigade was akin to the rural workplace, these infirmaries were the rural equivalent of the TB-treatment facilities set up by urban workplaces. Despite these initial efforts, anti-TB personnel in Songjiang did not consider their

---

9. The *Songjiang Health Gazetteer* does not list the reasons for the closure of these five facilities; however, given the timing, their closure might be due, in part, to the economic retrenchment following the Great Leap Forward.

network "complete" until the three levels of the CMS—county, township, and brigade—developed in the 1970s (Qian and Zhang 1985).

After the CMS reached maturity, each of the levels functioned in similar ways to the levels in the urban health-care system. The county TB prevention and treatment clinic was in charge of the entire county. It set goals and guided health workplaces to develop prevention and treatment work, trained doctors in commune-level pulmonary departments, and encouraged nurses to complete BCG immunization work. It supervised the township and village anti-TB group, the rural anti-TB group, a BCG group, and a statistical group. The county clinic had an outpatient department and an inpatient department with 50 beds and mostly treated severe cases (Y. Zhang 1989). When the county central hospital discovered TB patients, it generally transferred them to the county TB prevention and treatment clinic, which oversaw treatment.

Songjiang's attention to TB control continued, even as the CMS disintegrated in other parts of China. In the two towns and 19 villages in Songjiang county, there were 21 health facilities with pulmonary departments responsible for the discovery of and treatment management for TB patients in the late 1980s. Songjiang County also had 322 village health stations, with village doctors responsible for prevention and treatment. Village doctors also oversaw patient treatment management, making sure patients took their medicine and received repeat checkups on time. In this way, village doctors facilitated compliance with treatment regimens, much as workplace doctors worked with district TB prevention and treatment clinics in urban areas to ensure compliance. This three-tiered structure was used to facilitate declining disease. The trend continued well into the 1980s: between 1975 and 1986, case notifications declined 64 percent, mortality declined 70 percent, and prevalence declined more than 94 percent (Y. Zhang 1989). The next section will look in more depth at how Songjiang continued to develop rural health infrastructure into the 1990s.

While the decline of TB prevalence in rural Shanghai was not as pronounced as in urban areas in the 1980s, declining TB indicators in several rural counties suggest some continuity of service, and there are data to substantiate this notion. For example, one 1994 article by two Jiading County Tuberculosis Prevention and Treatment Clinic employees describes efforts to strengthen and solidify all three levels of the anti-TB network between 1985 and 1992. During this time, the township level—which had replaced the commune—played a particularly vital role in TB control. Each township-level health facility chose a pulmonologist to spend at least two days per week on anti-TB work. These doctors coordinated with personnel at both other levels of the rural health system. They supervised village doctors' anti-TB work, including BCG inoculations, and they also attended county-level meetings to discuss cases once every two weeks (Wang and Chen 2004). In Jiading County, registration of active cases of TB fell by more than 70 percent (from 75 to 22.4 per 100,000) between 1985 and 1992 (Wang and Chen 2004). While TB had been the seventh-leading cause of death in Jiading County in 1973 and 1980, by 1990, it disappeared from the list of the top 10 (Jiading Compilation Committee).

Change and Continuity in the Reform Era

China's post-1978 economic miracle was driven largely by rural industry. Nationally, output from rural enterprises grew 26 percent annually between 1978 and 1990, and the labor force engaged in township and village enterprises doubled (Oi 1999: 1). This dramatic growth also led to dramatic changes to rural entitlements. Within a few years of the onset of economic reform in 1978, most rural production brigades were dismantled, agricultural land was divided among village families, and the CMS's foundation collapsed in much of China. A survey conducted in 1985 showed that nationwide, CMS coverage plummeted from 90 percent to 5 percent. In 1989, coverage was estimated at only 4.8 percent (S. Wang 2004).

In Shanghai's rural counties, township and village enterprises (TVEs) continued to fund rural welfare services as they expanded throughout the 1980s (Cook 1999). Even at the beginning of the reform period, Shanghai's rural counties had a high level of industrialization compared to other parts of China. In 1977, Shanghai had just over 5,000 TVEs, which employed 550,000 workers and produced 2.1 billion RMB. These figures increased dramatically over the next decade. In 1988, Shanghai's rural counties had nearly 13,000 "industrial TVEs, 1.5 million workers, and 21.5 billion yuan of total output" (Buck 2012: 25). Shanghai's counties experienced a sevenfold increase of industrial output between 1980 and 1990. In 1986, collective enterprises including TVEs accounted for 93.5 percent of the gross income of all of Shanghai's rural enterprises. In townships with well-developed industries, government expenditures for public services consumed only a fraction of industrial revenues. In contrast, townships without strong industries could not meet their public service obligations in Shanghai or elsewhere in China. In Shanghai's counties, well-developed industries meant continued social provisions.

To turn more specifically to Songjiang, Philip Huang (1990) notes that industrial expansion ensured continued access to social services. Songjiang is farther from the urban core than Shanghai County, sitting immediately to its west. Until 1958, the county was part of Jiangsu Province. "Between 1962 and 1977, the municipal and county public finance bureaus provided 5.2 million yuan in interest free loans" to boost commune industries (Whiting 2001: 66). This investment led to development of the machinery, garment, and chemical industries, and by 1978, commune and brigade enterprises accounted for 42

142   *Tuberculosis Control and Institutional Change in Shanghai*

percent of GVIO. As the communes became townships and brigades became villages, industry continued to grow. In 1994, township enterprises accounted for 72 percent and village enterprises for nearly 26 percent of GVIO.

In Songjiang County, expansion of rural industries allowed several of the large village and township (乡镇) health facilities to also expand in the 1980s, 1990s, and beyond. For instance, Xinbin Town built a new 3,150-square-meter facility in 1986 (Yu 2011). This hospital had more than twice the square footage of the previous facility. It had 40 beds, 36 staff, and several departments, including internal medicine, surgery, and maternity. In 1998, an additional investment allowed the facility to expand its footprint by 13 percent, including a geriatric ward and 80 additional beds. But growth in the number of personnel did not always accompany facility development. The size of this facility would continue to expand over the next decade, to 4,187 square meters with 135 beds, but the number of staff declined from 49 in 1998 to 42 in 2006 (Yu 2011).

Other rural facilities in Songjiang also expanded in the 1980s and 1990s. The Xiaokunshan Township Hospital expanded its facilities by 350 square meters in 1991, and the hospital in the Gusong Administrative Region nearly doubled in size in 1992 (Yu and Liu 2012). The Xinqiao Township Hospital also expanded its area by 64 percent in 2002 (Q. Liu 2011). Each of these cases of infrastructure expansion occurred at the large village (乡) or town (镇) level, rather than at the grassroots (村) level, illustrating infrastructural improvements at the middle level of the rural health-care system, which did not receive as much attention when the CMS was in place.

At the grassroots level (村), the picture in Songjiang County is much more mixed, particularly with respect to maintenance of health personnel. The *Xinqiao Town Gazetteer* notes that the half-doctor-half-peasant model no longer met the growing needs of society, so the barefoot doctors went through additional training and took tests to become village doctors. In the 1980s, Xinqiao had 38 village doctors. In the 1990s, these village doctors received advanced training at Jiaotong University to allow them to meet the growing demands of society (Liu 2011). Some of Songjiang's rural towns, maintained their village doctors into the 1990s, but in others the number was dramatically reduced. For instance, Sheshan had 67 village doctors in 1985 and 70 in 1993, but in neighboring Tianma, the number of village doctors dropped from 54 in 1985 to 15 in 1993 (Liu and Yu 2012: 569). In 1985, Huayangqiao and Chedun Administrative Regions had 33 clinics, with 104 personnel. In 1998, Huayangqiao and Chedun had only 27 clinics with 58 personnel, 54 of whom had earned the village doctor certificate, and four of whom earned a sanitation worker's certificate (Zhao 2011a: 447). Thus, the number of doctors remaining was significantly reduced, but they were better credentialed. Reduction of personnel at the grassroots level actually matters little with respect to TB control because in the 1990s China implemented a 10-year TB control plan; under this plan, responsibility for treatment implementation shifted from the grassroots to a higher administrative level, but grassroots personnel were still sometimes enlisted to ensure Direct Observed Therapy, short-course (DOTS) compliance (Wang et al. 2007).

Shanghai County experienced changes in the training of rural health workers early in the Reform period. In 1985, Gong You-Long, deputy dean of Shanghai Medical College School of Public Health, visited Shanghai County to evaluate the changes to the rural health system. Gong had previously published on the county's rural health services and wanted to investigate changes in the Reform era. Gong and his collaborators discovered minimal attrition of BFDs to other professions. In 1980, there had been 751 BFDs, and in 1985, there were still 743 (Koplan et al. 1985). While some scholars feared that a more expensive, less egalitarian rural health system was replacing the CMS (V. W. Sidel and R. Sidel 1982; Henderson and Cohen 1984), this had not yet happened in Shanghai County as a result of initial reforms. At first, the primary changes were improvements; namely, increased certification and performance monitoring alleviated the problem of uneven training. The provincial level developed examinations, which BFDs needed to pass to be certified and continue to practice as "village doctors." As part of this credentialing system, the county funds for BFD training increased by 150 percent in 1982 (Koplan et al. 1985). The county vocational school also invited BFDs to take part in a full-time, one-year course or a part-time, two-year course taught via television.

These changes to the training structure at the village level occurred relatively early in the reform era, but increasing investment in rural health care at the township level throughout the 1980s suggests that leaders were adapting to the structural changes taking place. In 1989, each of Shanghai County's 14 villages and two townships had a hospital, but their facilities and personnel varied considerably. Interestingly, Hongqiao Commune, which was noted above as having a large population and a high population-to-BFD ratio in the early 1980s, made considerable investment in its township hospital in the 1980s. In 1989, Hongqiao had the largest township hospital in terms of square footage, with the largest number of beds and the second-largest number of staff, among the township and village hospitals in the county (Lü 1990: 40).

Some counties even began to develop policies to finance a new version of a cooperative medical system. For instance, in Fengxian County, the annual increase in medical fees led to financial losses and 27 percent of village cooperative medical services became paralyzed or disintegrated in the 1980s. Consequently, in June 1991, the county government published a policy on strengthening the rural cooperative medical system, which recommended taxing village enterprises to provide workers medical fees. In 1991, 11 villages invested 4.267 million RMB into the CMS. By the next year, the program had expanded to 19 villages, with an investment of 11.59 million RMB. In 1993, every village in the county had implemented a rural CMS plan in which it invested 17.45 million RMB. Between 1991 and 2001, investment in the CMS increased from 12 to 20 RMB per person, to 80 to 100 RMB per person; the investment by township and village enterprises increased from 40 to 60 RMB per person to 120 to 200 RMB per person, which brought the rural cooperative medical system to stability (J. Wang 2004). A similar "New Cooperative Medical System" would eventually be adopted throughout much of rural China in 2006.

Disease Control in a Former Rural District in the Twenty-First Century

To examine how the health system had changed in Shanghai's rural areas in recent years, I visited one of Shanghai's formerly rural counties. A contact in the District CDC quickly debunked my assumption that the health needs of Shanghai's rural residents had been well met by collective units in the 1970s: residents of this area "did not have work units" or the benefits associated with the work-unit system until after this former county was incorporated as an urban district, but they agreed that the health provisions and disease control functions between the rural and urban systems shared similar characteristics. My informant had arranged for me to see how disease control was being conducted in two contemporary work units in the former rural county, and they accompanied me on these visits on April 28, 2011. At each of the facilities, I spoke to personnel associated with on-site medical facilities. Both the case selection—the units were models for disease control—and the fact that members of the district CDC accompanied me ensured presentation of an idealized picture. Nevertheless, this visit served to highlight how health provision was being designed to allow people to interact with the health system in the places where they live and work.

We first visited the Strong Ox[10] conglomerate of seven factories that manufactured laptops in a high-tech park. They had a combined workforce of 68,000 workers, and at the time of our visit, they were in the process of expanding to 80,000. The workforce came from all over China. Most, including the management team, were on three-year contracts. Most were young adults and lived in dorms in the residential quarters on the perimeter of the compound, which had cafeterias and recreational facilities, such as basketball courts (Fieldnotes from April 2011). The close proximity of the residential quarters to the factories resembled that of some former urban work units. Our visit coincided with a change in shifts, so we could see thousands of young people in work uniforms walking between the residential quarters and the factory.

---

10. A pseudonym.

Building and Maintaining the Tuberculosis Control Network   145

The health and disease control provisions of this contemporary factory illustrate interventions similar to those made under the WUS. The company employs 10 doctors—one for each factory and three for the residential quarters—as well as 33 nurses, who worked in shifts, so workers had access to a health-care provider on a 24-hour basis. Annual physicals were offered to all workers, but unlike under the work-unit system, workers are not required to participate. Consequently, only 70–80 percent of workers actually did. By employing health personnel and maintaining on-site clinics, the conglomerate helped to keep costs low, but since the vast majority of the workers were young, health costs were low anyway. The medical staff sometimes do outreach, including providing public service announcements in cafeterias and holding classes on topics like mental health. The compound also has a facility where they isolate suspected cases during disease outbreaks.

After leaving the factory, we visited a health clinic in the university district, which illustrated typical health provision for university students in several ways. Most of the school's 10,000 students were located on this satellite campus, rather than the campus closer to the urban core. All students on both campuses, as well as throughout Shanghai, had a standardized form of health insurance, which had been available to students in Shanghai since 2007. If they were sick or injured in a nonemergency situation, students were expected to first visit the school clinic to be referred to a more advanced facility as necessary. The staff at the facility we visited pointed out that services at their facility are subsidized: students have to pay only 40 RMB for a checkup, but chest X-rays alone actually cost their clinic 60–80 RMB to provide. Thus, this clinic provides preventive care and serves as the gatekeeper for students (and staff) to more advanced medical facilities. Through their provision of health services, this and other universities might be viewed as maintaining the types of services offered in urban areas under the work-unit system.

This university's disease prevention efforts were strong and sought to compensate for students whose immune systems are compromised by stress. Students there actively participate in the production of preventive health materials. As an example, 78 students entered a contest sponsored by the CDC to design public health materials for International Tuberculosis Awareness Day in March 2011. The winning design was used in CDC materials throughout the municipality. According to my respondent, Shanghai sees only around 20 TB cases annually among its 80,000 university students. Of the cases, most are among second- and third-year students; however, the medical staff pointed out a challenging phenomenon they occasionally encounter. Students are required to have a physical examination when they take the university entrance exam (高考) the summer before they enter the university. Yet, on rare occasions, freshmen are found to have advanced cases of active TB when they begin school only a few months later.

Since it would be impossible to develop an advanced case of tuberculosis in just a few months, this suggests that these students provided fraudulent documents— perhaps they submitted someone else's health test results, rather than their own—when they took the college entrance exam. This example illustrates the incredible pressure that students feel to pass the exam. Indeed, students' health is an occasional casualty of this high-pressure, test-based education system. The contest to design health materials was created to help students reprioritize their health. Students participated, much as they had in SATA's essay contest during the Japanese Occupation. Thus, a few even became active participants in health promotion.

During my visit to this formerly rural county, I was well aware that I was being shown model units, just as foreign delegations were taken on "carefully choreographed" visits to the Chinese countryside in the 1970s (Zhou 2020: 246). Nevertheless, this visit highlighted the way health insurance service provision and disease control was fairly comprehensive for some contemporary residents of Shanghai's formerly rural areas in 2011. In contrast to other places in China, this district saw investment in a high-tech park, which attracted companies that provided benefits packages, including health care. Likewise, this district committed to infrastructure advancement and set up a university district, which attracted satellite campuses of several established institutions in downtown Shanghai. These two workplaces illustrate adaptation in the reform era, a topic that will be explored in more depth in the following chapter.

Conclusion

Following the revolutionary institutional change of collectivization in the 1950s and 1960s, Shanghai's rural counties established a production-brigade-based health-care system. Given that the production brigade was the administrative equivalent of the work unit in rural areas, this system was the functional equivalent of the work-unit system, and there are certainly parallels with respect to health provision. To a great extent, the rural CMS relied upon paraprofessional health workers to execute preventive programming and curative services for the most common diseases, including TB. Production brigade members could be referred to higher-level health facilities if a condition or disease was beyond the scope of the training of rural health personnel, and costs incurred when visiting higher-level facilities were covered by the rural production brigade. This three-tiered system also facilitated TB control. Rural areas throughout China established and used similar rural health systems between 1968 and the dismantling of collective agriculture in the early 1980s.

While the 1980s dismantling of the rural production brigades led to collapse of the CMS in many areas of China, this research suggests that Shanghai's formerly rural counties adapted to this dynamic situation. Rural Shanghai's growing industrial sector allowed for expansion of mid-level rural health facilities in some rural counties. At the grassroots level, some of the former barefoot doctors received advanced training, were credentialed as village doctors, and continued to provide care beyond the 1980s; however, their numbers were reduced in places. The chapter also illustrates that some formerly rural areas in Shanghai saw such heavy investment that they were able to provide coverage nearly as complete as under the work-unit system. These findings cannot necessarily be generalized beyond Shanghai, because Shanghai's rural industries were more developed. Rural health provision and TB control in Shanghai's rural areas was better than TB control in rural areas of most other provinces, both before and after the dismantling of the rural production brigades. Peasants elsewhere in China were never served as well as were those in Shanghai. Many places in China saw a severe collapse of the brigade-level health stations in the 1980s, and the New Cooperative Medical System was not created for 20 years.

Part III

Post-Work-Unit Era, 1992–2011

6

Dismantling of the Work-Unit System and Challenges to Tuberculosis Control in Shanghai, 1992–2011

On December 24, 2010, I interviewed a 20-year-old TB patient who had just flown home to China from the Canadian university where she was studying. This patient was diagnosed after she had been in Canada for her first year of school. She had been coughing for 3–4 months and saw a doctor only after she returned home to China. She was diagnosed in July 2009 and had been taking a standard course of TB drugs for 17 months. She had never seen a Canadian doctor about her illness; instead, she bought all of her medicine in Shanghai and took it with her when she went to Canada each semester. She had follow-up appointments only upon returning to China between semesters. Given her family's wealth, this young woman had a lot of choices regarding both her education and health care. Her mother had an "average" salary in a state-owned enterprise, but her father worked at a private company, so they did not find the first-line TB drugs particularly expensive. Since Shanghai is the closest international airport to her home in Hefei, it was convenient for this young woman to see the doctor in Shanghai before returning to Anhui Province for the winter holiday. This example illustrates how convenient it is for those with means to seek care at top treatment facilities in Shanghai (TB Interview 22).

Her experience contrasted sharply with that of another patient I had interviewed nine days prior. That patient, a 36-year-old homemaker from the countryside near Anhui Province, had been in treatment since January 2005, almost six years. Li Chunying had an elementary education, and started working as a manual laborer at age 17. She had not worked since giving birth to her children—a 13-year-old son and a 6-year-old daughter—and she self-reported that her health knowledge was fairly low. In fact, because she did not understand why taking a full course of antibiotics was important when she was first being treated for TB, she had stopped taking her medicines against her doctor's orders; thus, if she had originally had a drug-susceptible strain, it had transformed into the drug-resistant strain she was now battling. While there was no way to know whether she had acquired resistance or had originally been infected with a drug-resistant strain, her treatment had involved numerous medications and three hospital stays. Her family paid the entire cost, including several hundred RMB per month for medications during her early treatment period. Medicines to combat resistant strains of TB are much more expensive, and she insisted on buying hers in Shanghai because she was concerned about the quality of medication in the countryside. She remembers that they spent 30,000 RMB the first time she was hospitalized for a month, and she had two subsequent hospitalizations of two weeks each. She had no idea how much total money her immediate family had spent, but she knew that they were in debt to several relatives. When she sought reimbursement, less than 10 percent of her costs had been covered (TB Interview 11).

These vignettes represent opposite ends of the spectrum of both disease complexity and care options available to contemporary TB patients in China. While patients were once geographically constrained to the health facilities that serviced their work units, patients now have choices. Anyone can travel to receive care as long as they can pay for those medical services. While some patients, such as the 20-year-old student, whose infection was responsive to first-line drugs, find these expenses trivial, patients with more complicated infections may end up in debt or depleting their savings so much that they compromise future life chances.

This chapter illustrates the complexity of TB control, following the major structural changes that occurred beginning in the 1990s. The chapters above have demonstrated that the story of TB control in China from the 1950s through the 1980s was one of gains against the disease. In the 1990s, some alarming trends emerged. Among them was stagnation of the number of cases being identified as a fraction of estimated total cases (Wang, Liu, and Chin 2007). This meant that persons with active disease were not being identified or treated, so TB was continuing to spread. Another alarming trend was the disproportionate number of drug-resistant cases. Around 2005, China was estimated to have only 15 percent of global TB cases but more than 30 percent of the burden of drug-resistant cases (Zhu et al. 2017). Both of these trends relate to declining access to health care. In some cases, TB was not being found because sufferers did not seek care for their illness. In other cases, persons with disease did not complete the full treatment course, leading to a rise in drug-resistant strains. This chapter demonstrates that the dismantling of the urban work-unit system was a major cause of faltering TB control.

Fundamental Institutional Change: Dismantling of the Work-Unit System

Four primary trends accompanied the shift from the planned economy to socialism with market characteristics: privatization, restructuring of enterprises to become profit oriented, elimination of permanent employment, and large-scale migration. Each of these trends represents a major structural change, and each has implications for disease control. The 1990s witnessed the growth of private enterprises and privatization or closure of numerous state-owned and collective enterprises. The central government prohibited large private enterprise until the late 1980s, but quite a few private enterprises arose alongside public ones. After 1992, privatization began to displace public ownership. As Mary Gallagher argues, "By the mid-1990s, it had become clear that SOE reform without privatization had reached a dead end" (2005: 134). The government ordered small- and medium-sized SOEs to be privatized. Nationally, the share of urban jobs in SOEs and collective-owned enterprises (COEs) fell from 76 percent in 1995, to 41 percent in 2000, to 27 percent in 2005 (Park and Cai 2011). In Shanghai, there were 2.1 million workers in state-owned industrial enterprises in 1992. Within five years, that number fell by nearly half, and by 2002 it fell to 384,700, a mere 18 percent of the 1992 figure (*Shanghai Statistical Yearbook* Editorial Committee 2004). Numbers of workers in Shanghai's collective-owned enterprises dropped 84 percent, from 421,100 in 1993 to 38,500 in 2003 (*Shanghai Statistical Yearbook* Editorial Committee 2004). While employment in manufacturing SOEs and COEs declined, employment in private enterprises, including manufacturing, service, and finance, increased.

Unsurprisingly, areas of Shanghai that had the most industry were hit especially hard by privatization. For example, in heavily industrialized Yangpu District, 154 factories closed by 2003 (*Shanghai Yangpu District Gazetteer* Compilation Committee 2009). While a dozen of these factories left the city or moved to industrial districts on the outskirts of Shanghai, the majority stopped doing business or closed their doors entirely. Common reasons for closure included bankruptcy and making way for new residential compounds. More than 30 of the factories closed to enable housing construction. For example, the Shanghai Construction Machinery Factory, which employed 2,000 workers, closed to make space for new dormitories at Fudan University (*Shanghai Yangpu District Gazetteer* Compilation Committee 2009). The 154 SOEs that closed in Yangpu varied considerably in size, but the closures affected at least 146,500 people.

A second change that occurred throughout China in the 1990s was the restructuring of remaining state-owned enterprises to be profit oriented. With growing competition between SOEs and private enterprises, which did not always provide generous benefits, the work-unit model was no longer sustainable. To remain competitive, SOEs had to shed welfare benefits, including health provisions. As welfare benefits were cut, the socialized, centralized state-responsibility model transformed back into the privatized, ad-hoc responsibility model that had existed prior to the 1950s creation of the work-unit system. Wage payments are now the only remaining responsibility of many workplaces to their workers.

In the 1990s, permanent employment also ended in favor of more unstable casual employment. Large-scale layoffs from state-owned and collective enterprises occurred as these institutions closed or were restructured in the late 1990s and early 2000s. According to official data, between 1998 and 2002, 25 million layoffs occurred in urban China (Bramall 2009). Following SOE reforms, the remaining state-owned firms and the increasing number of private enterprises hired workers, often for low wages with few benefits (Andreas 2012). Scholars of labor in China have studied how this trend led to a rise of informal and precarious labor (Park and Cai 2011; Lin 2015; Swider 2015). This change occurred in both urban areas and in the remaining rural industries, which slashed wages to remain competitive.

The fourth trend of the 1990s followed directly from the move toward unstable, casual employment: the beginning of large-scale migration. As is the case in other global locations, trying to determine the size of the migrant population is extremely difficult for several reasons. Among them, migrants might be undercounted because their official registration remains elsewhere or they are informally employed. According to official estimates, the number of rural-to-urban migrants nationally was estimated to be 20 million in 1990, around 100 million in 2000, and more than 220 million in 2010 (Lu and Xia 2016). In Shanghai, the aggregate population of rural migrants was estimated at 10 million at the time of the 2010 census (Chan 2012). Many of these migrants were drawn to emerging industries. In 2003, an estimated 734,700 migrants in Shanghai worked in manufacturing, 555,300 in construction, 394,600 in commercial services, and around 200,000 each in agriculture, domestic service, and the food and beverage industry (*Shanghai Statistical Yearbook* Editorial Committee 2004).

The population of rural migrants who live in urban areas but do not possess urban residence permits is often called the "floating population" (流动人口) because there is the perception that they are only temporary workers who frequently return to their sending areas. In actuality, many of these individuals do not float between receiving and sending areas very regularly; they might not have a residence permit for their receiving area, but they are in the cities to stay. Throughout the 1990s, migrants' access to public services, such as schools and health care, was limited. While some scholars have questioned whether residence permits have declined in significance, the consensus seems to be that migrants' status as urban citizens remains contested (Solinger 1999;

Chan and Buckingham 2008; Zhan 2011). Certainly, systemic barriers to services have declined in recent years, but many of Shanghai's migrants still face the same sorts of quality-of-life and health-care access challenges as do migrants in other global cities. For example, until the relatively recent increased access to media and labor organizations, few migrants were aware of their rights. Consequently, they often worked long hours for little pay. Likewise, many lived in substandard, crowded housing, making them more vulnerable to disease exposure. They also face challenges to accessing care, such as lack of time, money, and transportation, or language barriers, since many are most comfortable in a dialect other than standard Mandarin (Chen et al. 2013). Thus, unequal access to resources might affect these individuals at any stage of the disease, from infection to death.

These four trends interrelated closely. Privatization and restructuring meant shedding benefits and ending permanent employment in favor of more unstable, casual employment, "dismantling the iron rice bowl" (Leung 1994; Gallagher, Lee, and Kuruvilla 2011; Andreas 2012). This new situation led to large-scale migration. These changing economic and demographic trends paired with reduced investment in health and public health have made for a challenging disease-control situation, as the trends map onto the factors that have contributed to globally resurgent TB. Migration is itself one of the factors that has contributed to resurgent TB; people are drawn to perceived opportunities but find themselves in a precarious situation, often with limited access to health resources. Changes to health and public health systems also contributed to globally resurgent TB, as health care became available to some but not to all. The next section looks more in depth at changes to the health system before turning to fundamental changes in the TB control system.

Changes to the Chinese Health System

During the work-unit era, the Chinese government was heavily invested in the health sector. This began to change with economic reform. Much of the most dramatic changes with respect to health spending occurred in the 1990s, which increased as a percent of GDP; however, government health spending as a proportion of GDP declined, while private spending increased. The central government's share of health spending as a percentage of total health expenditure went from 36 percent in the 1980s to 15 percent in 2000 (Tang, Brixi, and Bekedam 2014). Throughout the 1980s and 1990s, the collective share of health spending also declined. During these two decades, the proportion of health spending covered by collectives, such as rural production brigades and other work units, dropped from 44 percent to 24.5 percent. Conversely, the proportion of health spending borne by individual families increased, as individuals were expected to make up the deficit. By 2000, the share of health spending borne by individuals

156

had increased to more than 60 percent (S. Wang 2004). Indeed, the model under which work units picked up the majority of health-care costs had disappeared, but in the past decade, the government sought to replace lost benefits to correct the access challenges my respondents and neighbors faced around 2010.

Changes to health infrastructure

As described above, while the work-unit system was fully in place, there was a three-tiered medical system, with grassroots clinics throughout the city (and surrounding counties) in Shanghai. Throughout the 1980s, the number of health-care institutions in both urban and rural areas of Shanghai continued to rise (Figure 6.2). Many of these clinics were workplace based. They provided primary health care at very little cost, and their users often only went to higher-level facilities upon referral when they could not be served in the local clinics. In 1990, the number of health-care institutions in Shanghai peaked at 7,690 and then began to decline. Some schools and a few remaining factories still had clinics, but the number of these facilities declined greatly until 2003, the same year as the SARS epidemic. At that time, there were only 2,319 health-care institutions in Shanghai, less than one-third of the number that had existed in 1990 (*Shanghai Statistical Yearbook* Editorial Committee 2017). Not surprisingly, areas of the city with numerous workplace-based clinics were deeply affected by this change. For example, closure of grassroots clinics hit Yangpu District hard: in 1990, Yangpu had a total of 429 healthcare facilities, including 377 factory clinics (*Shanghai Yangpu District Gazetteer* Compilation Committee 2009). In 2007, the total number of health institutions in Yangpu was just 174 (*Shanghai Statistical Yearbook* Editorial Committee 2008).

Community health centers were set up in Shanghai in the early 2000s to partially replace workplace clinics. CHCs were expected to provide many of the functions once undertaken by work-unit clinics, such as providing care for chronic conditions like hypertension and diabetes. One goal of these centers was to stem the tide of individuals going to higher, municipal-level facilities; however, because Chinese citizens had a choice about where to receive health care, many skipped the step of referral and went straight to municipal-level hospitals, even for minor illnesses. There was also the perception that CHCs had lower prices because of lower quality of care (Provider 11; Yang and Yang 2009; Qian et al. 2010; Bhattacharyya et al. 2011; Wang et al. 2012). Consequently, these facilities were initially underutilized and did not really relieve the burden of overloaded municipal-level hospitals.

Other scholars have characterized the post-SARS years as an era of recovery for public health in China (Wang et al. 2019). Indeed, in 2004, China enacted a Revised Law on the Prevention and Control of Infectious Diseases, and as Figure

Figure 6.1: Number of health-care institutions in Shanghai, 1978–2016

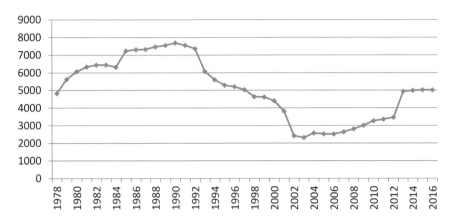

Source: *Shanghai Statistical Yearbook 2017.*

6.1 illustrates, Shanghai saw an increase in health facilities. In 2009, the Chinese government intensified health reforms to improve the efficiency of the systems. Among the changes it envisioned was establishing a more widespread primary health-care system, where doctors at CHCs in urban areas and township health centers in rural areas would serve as gatekeepers, managing referrals to higher-level facilities (Wang et al. 2012; Yip et al. 2012). However, scholars have pointed out that provision of community health care lagged behind the development of infrastructure in two regards. First, the public needed to embrace the idea of primary, community-based medicine more fully. Second, trained personnel, including general practitioners and nurses, were needed to staff them (Wang et al. 2012; Yip et al. 2012). These problems presented challenges for cost and efficiency to the overall urban and rural health systems; however, their development largely does not affect TB control. The CHCs may help to oversee adherence to TB treatment, but they do not have the authority to set the treatment course. Instead, as will be described below, they are required to send suspected cases to district-level facilities (Provider 11).

Changes to health financing

When the work-unit system was in place, urban residents were covered by one of two health insurance systems, the labor insurance system or government insurance system. Under this system, controlling hospital costs was a goal because treatment costs were borne by the workplace. As described in Chapters 4 and 5, in both urban and rural areas, the workplace or brigade clinic played a key role in controlling health-care costs. Health workers held preventive educational programs, for both TB and other ailments. Health workers also helped to monitor the health of their fellow laborers, and workplaces paid for regular checkups. This was done to help detect ailments early so they could be treated at the local level. The decline of primary health institutions has led to rising costs. Since members of the population have had more choice regarding where to receive care, many have sought care in higher-level facilities. As the vignettes at the beginning of the chapter illustrate, in some cases, persons even travel to the most developed cities, like Shanghai, in their quest to find the best treatment.

With declines in state funding of health institutions themselves, higher-level health facilities, such as district and municipal hospitals, were in no hurry to control costs. From the perspective of health-care institutions such as hospitals, governmental disinvestment in the health sector, paired with the government-imposed system of price regulation, led to perverse incentives to recover costs. This has been true in both urban and rural areas. Pharmaceutical sales and fees from the use of high-tech equipment have been used in an attempt to recover costs (Deng, Wilkes, and Bloom 1997; Blumenthal and Hsiao 2005). These changes explain part of the increase in health spending, much of which has been passed on to the consumer.

Increasing costs to the consumer led to several unfortunate trends in care seeking, some of which became evident after the collapse of the rural CMS more widely. The first trend was delays in care seeking. Persons with flu-like symptoms choose to self-medicate rather than seek care in the health system due to worries about cost. A second, similar trend is patients seeking an early discharge from hospitals or other care facilities owing to an inability to pay. A third trend is individuals who choose to completely forego care. These trends have been well documented (Henderson et al. 1994; S. Wang 2004; Tang, Brixi, and Bekedam 2014). From the perspective of TB control or newly emerging infections, these factors created a dangerous situation. Foregoing care or delaying treatment means that the disease continues to spread, and stopping care in the middle can lead to drug-resistant strains.

In the 1990s, several cities in China began to implement new urban health insurance schemes to replace the declining LIS and GIS systems. In Shanghai, this scheme began in 1996, when both employees and employers began contributing to health accounts. Under this system, employees contribute a small percentage of their annual salary to a health insurance account. Likewise, employers contribute a small percentage of their total wage bill to a municipally pooled health insurance fund. When individuals become sick or injured, they first rely on the funds in their individual account to cover costs. Urban residents must draw upon these funds or pay out of pocket until the expenses from a given illness total 10 percent of the average annual wage for the city of Shanghai. Thereafter, pooled

Dismantling of the Work-Unit System and Challenges to Tuberculosis Control   159

funds kick in (Ducket 2004). But pooled municipal funds do not meet the entire remaining cost of catastrophic illnesses. The cap on pooled funds is four times the average annual salary for Shanghai. Once the cap is exceeded, patients and their families are expected to pay any additional costs. Naturally, these expenses affect poor, laid-off workers and unskilled migrant workers more than they do wealthy individuals, who have more disposable income.

While this program began in 1996, by 1999, only 5 million of Shanghai's labor force of 8.4 million (or 60 percent) had joined the scheme. Nationally, just over half (56 percent) of urban residents were covered by some form of medical insurance at the turn of the century, but numerous individuals, for instance, temporary workers and those in the informal sector, were completely excluded from municipal schemes (S. Wang 2004). These individuals included migrants, such as domestic helpers, many of whom never receive any sort of work contract.

Residents of most of Shanghai's rural areas began to be covered under the municipal insurance program in the 1990s, as the rural counties were incorporated into urban districts, but residents of most rural areas in China remained outside of urban systems. As noted in Chapter 5, in rural areas of China, cooperative medical system coverage reached more than 90 percent of the rural population by 1980; however, in the 1980s, the dismantling of production brigades prompted disinvestment, leaving most rural residents throughout China to fend for themselves until the New Cooperative Medical System began to be implemented in 2006.

Chinese citizens have raised objections to these reforms. Since 2000, tens of thousands of medical protests (医闹) have erupted throughout China on an annual basis (Kerrigan 2018; Tu 2019). These protests have attracted media scrutiny and prompted additional reforms. Wide-scale health reforms in 2009 attempted to improve insurance coverage for urban and rural residents throughout the country. By 2011, 92 percent of the population was covered by an urban or rural insurance scheme (Yip et al. 2012). However, coverage initially came with shallow benefits. For instance, basic medical insurance for urban residents (implemented nationwide in 2003) and the NCMS initially only covered some inpatient services. Recipients still had to pay many associated costs, such as deductibles and copayments, resulting in more than half of these expenditures being born by individuals (Yip et al. 2012). Costs borne by the individual for outpatient services were even greater, as least initially. My interviews took place at a time that this program was beginning to ramp up; yet, as data from my interviews with TB patients illustrates, patients had varying levels of coverage during their illness. The situation has continued to improve in the past decade, but there remain gaps between people's right to health care and the actualization of this right.

Fundamental Change and Tuberculosis Control

Changes to TB control infrastructure

Under the work-unit system, both urban and rural residents of Shanghai were well served by the TB control network, which made full use of the three-tiered health systems. This program emphasized identifying cases early in workplaces to help control treatment costs. Between 1992 and 1998, a municipal TB control facility remained in place, but the TB prevention and treatment clinics in urban districts and rural counties closed. The doctors and nurses who had been employed at the district prevention and treatment clinics joined other district-level facilities, such as chronic disease prevention hospitals or central district hospitals. Most districts reduced the number of personnel dedicated to TB control. For instance, a retired doctor I interviewed who had worked throughout this period said that her workplace, a district-level TB clinic, had 12 doctors and 18 nurses prior to 1992, but after 1992 had only 5 doctors in the TB prevention and treatment department (Provider 30).

Starting in 1998, Shanghai again developed a standardized TB policy, with distinct roles for the three levels of health facilities. This policy is under the direction of the Shanghai Center for Disease Control, which was established in 1998. The Shanghai CDC modeled itself after the US CDC and was the first CDC in China. Its establishment responded to both changing disease patterns and structural changes—such as the dismantling of SOEs and the ensuing crisis in preventive health (Peng et al. 2003). Within the three tiers of responsibility, the municipal-level CDC guides TB policy and maintains records of the number and status of cases throughout the city. District-level branches of the CDC undertake some of the tasks once handled by district prevention and treatment clinics, providing educational programming in schools and deploying mobile X-ray units to workplaces when requested. At the same time, designated district-level treatment hospitals set the course of treatment for individual patients. Neighborhood-level community health centers have partially replaced clinics in individual workplaces—they oversee patient compliance with treatment regimens, as workplaces once did—but unlike when the work-unit system was in place, patients can choose to go to higher-level facilities if they have the ability to pay. Thus, sometimes lower-level clinics are unaware of cases that might have previously fallen under their purview.

Problems with DOTS

Following the World Health Organization's elevation of tuberculosis to a global health emergency in 1993, it increased promotion of the DOTS model, which

Dismantling of the Work-Unit System and Challenges to Tuberculosis Control   161

came to dominate TB control globally in the 1990s. This program has five basic components (WHO 1999). First, the program requires political commitment and sustained financing for any country signing up. Second, it emphasizes case detection through sputum smear testing.[1] Third, it requires patients to undergo a standardized treatment course during which they receive supervision from health professionals. Patients with bacterial-positive results on the sputum smear test are reimbursed for the cost of a six-month course of standardized TB medicines. Fourth, governments are asked to ensure and manage a supply of effective TB antibiotics. Finally, the program requires governments to develop an effective, centralized reporting system for monitoring and evaluating the program's impact.

In the 1980s and 1990s, the WHO encouraged numerous developing countries to replace their existing TB control programs with the low-cost DOTS strategy. DOTS has been very successful in many developing countries; however, some scholars and practitioners believe that its entry into national health systems of some middle-income countries was a technocratic imposition. For instance, in his 2001 dissertation, "Reform and Resistance in Post-Soviet Tuberculosis Control," Gene Bukhman argues that the DOTS program was not as good as tuberculosis control during the Soviet era. Bukhman claims that DOTS was a "Volkswagen," not a "Rolls Royce"—that is, the program was a one-size-fits-all model that could be quickly scaled up to cover a large population rather than custom made. Bukhman's perspectives on the former Soviet Union provide some important insights for China, where a number of deficiencies with DOTS may have contributed to its challenges in TB control. These deficiencies include coverage exclusions, problems with the case-finding model, and reimbursement difficulties.

Coverage exclusions apply to both limitations on types of TB and geographical areas or populations. Only smear-positive, drug-susceptible, pulmonary TB was covered.[2] This meant that patients with smear-negative TB and extrapulmonary TB (such as lymph and bone TB) were not covered. Additionally, and crucially important, until recent years, the DOTS program covered only the standard first-line course of TB drugs and not second- and third-line drugs. Consequently, those with drug-resistant strains necessarily incurred treatment costs (Provider 6). With funding from a World Bank loan, this program was put into place in some areas of China in 1992, but DOTS did not include as many services or medication options as had been covered under the work-unit system.

---

1. Chest X-rays were the gold standard for TB case detection in China and elsewhere in the world in the 1950s and 1960s. By the 1980s, the sputum smear test had become the gold standard for identifying cases of active TB in many parts of the world.
2. Smear-positive TB tests suggest a high bacterial load and likelihood of transmission.

In terms of geographical exclusions, DOTS was initially implemented in only 13 of China's provinces, municipalities, and autonomous regions, but it was quickly scaled up to cover 90 percent of the population (Chen et al. 2002). Shanghai municipality was not initially included in DOTS, but its districts did adopt some of the DOTS policy recommendations. Most individual districts opted to provide a standard six-month course of treatment drugs to their residents, but there was variation in what was provided among districts. Because Shanghai was China's richest province, treatment costs were assumed not to be a barrier for most individuals (China Tuberculosis Control Collaboration 2004). However, while Shanghai was China's wealthiest province in terms of per-capita GDP, the dual phenomena of mass layoffs and mass in-migration during the 1990s meant that income inequality was growing. As was the case before the work-unit system was put into place, those with the least income to pay for treatment were most likely to be at risk of developing TB because of their living and working conditions.

The most important geographical exclusion was that through 2003 migrants could only receive treatment in their place of official residence. They were excluded from the program in their receiving areas. This meant that migrants had to travel back to their sending areas to seek care when they had an active infectious disease, which would mean months of lost income. The alternative to this was to pay out of pocket. Starting in 2004–2006 cities with large and increasing migrant populations worked to expand coverage, but some coverage exclusions remained.

In addition to coverage exclusions, the DOTS case-finding model, passive case finding, is arguably inferior to the models used under the work-unit system. Passive case finding rests on the assumption that the public will recognize disease symptoms themselves and voluntarily report to disease-control facilities. As the number of cases identified declined, Shanghai began to embrace this international recommendation and move away from annual chest X-rays. Workplaces were still supposed to require health checks—and many still did when employees were hired—but as the 1990s progressed and SOEs fell into crisis, many did not have the money to pay for annual physicals. Consequently, employers' requests for visits from mobile X-ray vehicles have declined (Providers 6, 12, 20, 30, and 34). The move from active to passive case finding represented a big change from the work-unit era, when health checks were given annually in large work units. Passive case finding is effective in an area where the population has received regular exposure to health educational programming but less effective in a heterogeneous population with uneven health educational backgrounds. In an area with large-scale in-migration, like Shanghai, education backgrounds among the population are certainly uneven.

Problems with care were twofold. First was the problem of where patients could receive care. Designated hospitals for providing TB care were often not as

Dismantling of the Work-Unit System and Challenges to Tuberculosis Control   163

conveniently located as workplace clinics had been. Consequently, patients could choose to receive care at the district-level facility that is either closest to their home or their workplace, but more commuting was inevitably involved. This raised questions of time, money, and the potential of infecting others on public transportation. Second, compliance to treatment regimens was not monitored as well as it used to be. Treatment was managed by personnel from district hospitals, rather than the combined effort of district and workplace doctors, which had been relatively effective during the work-unit era. The present program's emphasis on Directly Observed Therapy is meant to alleviate compliance problems; however, as the second vignette at the beginning of the chapter indicates, some patients do not understand the importance of taking the full course of antibiotics when they start to feel better.

Finally, DOTS has a number of reimbursement problems. Reimbursement does not cover all costs associated with illness, but over the years Shanghai has expanded the program to cover more of patients' expenses. Transportation costs were not covered when the program began, but they were subsequently added. The program covers smear tests but not CT scans, which doctors might use to monitor how the disease is progressing in the lungs. The program does not cover Chinese medicines, which are often prescribed as part of treatment to help alleviate side effects of the standard DOTS drugs and are more expensive than the DOTS medicines. Finally, reimbursement procedures cannot be undertaken until the six-month course of drugs was complete. As is demonstrated in the evidence from some of my interviews, procedures were also unnecessarily complicated (TB Interviews 8 and 24).

A Spectrum of Coverage in TB Care

How has the healthcare access of individuals been affected by such dramatic changes to the urban health infrastructure, urban insurance programs, and the TB control programs? Have individuals been able to obtain care at a reasonable cost? To what extent has cost been a factor in whether and when to seek care? I conducted intensive, in-person interviews in Mandarin Chinese with 45 tuberculosis patients being treated at a municipal-level facility between December 2010 and July 2011. These patients were identified through respondent-driven sampling. For the interviews, I targeted individuals who began working when the work-unit system was still in place to allow my respondents to contrast the types of care they received under both systems; however, I found that young individuals with concerns about how the disease might compromise their future were particularly eager to talk about their experience. Age was a critical variable in my analysis. Those who were over the age of 35 would have been at least 20 years old in 1995 and consequently were likely to have had experience working

164   *Tuberculosis Control and Institutional Change in Shanghai*

under the work-unit system. Patients' varying ages gave them diverse perspectives on how transformations of the economic and health systems affected access to care. Table 6.1 presents an aggregated snapshot of the basic demographic characteristics of my sample, and Appendix B provides the basic demographic information—gender, age, place of residence, and occupation—for each respondent.

Table 6.1: Tuberculosis patient interviewees' characteristics

Gender	Male	Female
	20	25
Age	Older than 35	Younger than 35
	19	26
Socioeconomic class*	Middle class or small business owner	Working class or working poor
	27 (22 white collar + 5 small business owners)	18
Place of residence	Shanghai	Outside Shanghai
	21	24

* Socioeconomic class distinctions are based on education level (college vs. noncollege) or position with respect to ownership or the means of production. Small business owners and managers are included as part of the middle class.

As Table 6.1 illustrates, interviewees included 24 people who came to Shanghai just for the purpose of seeing a doctor. Some of these patients came to Shanghai because they had a more complicated infection of drug-resistant or extrapulmonary TB. Consequently, they are slightly overrepresented in my sample. Within my sample six patients (or 13.33 percent) were being treated for MDR TB, while the actual number of patients with MDR among TB patients in China is approximately 1 in 10. The majority of patients who traveled for treatment researched online and elected to come to Shanghai because they believed they could get the best possible treatment. These patients tended to be internet savvy and consequently a bit younger. Those from outside Shanghai had a mean age of 34, while those who lived in Shanghai had a mean age of 38. While we might expect patients with enough means to travel for health care to be relatively wealthy, as the chapter's opening vignettes illustrate, this was not always the case.

The rest of the chapter examines the health care access of 14 TB patients with differing means and levels of health insurance coverage, as well as differing levels of illness complexity. The interviews uncovered a spectrum of coverage based upon whether and where individual workers were employed.

Dismantling of the Work-Unit System and Challenges to Tuberculosis Control   165

Best access: Wealthy individuals who travel distances to receive care

Persons who were employed in lucrative private enterprises (or who had family employed in lucrative private enterprises) were sometimes willing to travel great distances to seek care, regardless of cost. The university student in the chapter's opening vignette was a good example of this sort of patient. Since the father had made money in the private sector, this family had a lot of choices regarding both the daughter's education and her healthcare. Fortunately, this student was the only person I interviewed who admitted to traveling on a long-haul flight when she had an active case of infectious disease, but two of my other respondents fell into the category of opting to fly a distance to receive care.

A second patient who flew to receive care was a 37-year-old manager from a major international hotel group. He had worked for 17 years, including 13 in food hygiene management. He was originally from Guangdong, but his company moved him to a different location every two to three years, so he had lived in several Chinese cities. At the time of our interview, he was based in Hohhot, but he traveled back to Shanghai for his follow-up appointment each year because he had been living in Shanghai when he was diagnosed with a lung cavity four years previously. He had surgery on the cavity and stayed in the hospital for a week. Fortunately, his illness turned out to be TB, rather than cancer, and he took first-line TB drugs. His employer provided health insurance, which covered a good portion of his estimated 100,000 RMB (approximately US$15,000) in expenses, most of which was incurred during the acute stage of the infection. Since he relocated from Shanghai, most of his considerable travel expenses were not covered (TB Interview 44). He was not worried about out-of-pocket expenses because he wanted to keep seeing the doctor that he trusted.

Like the hotel manager, a 38-year-old businesswoman was not concerned about the expenses she incurred while traveling to receive care. She had gotten her start working in a hair salon, from the age of 15 to 23. More recently, she sold Dell computers, which had taken her from her home in Wenzhou to Sichuan. After being diagnosed with tuberculosis seven months prior to our interview, she had taken first-line antibiotics, which she estimated cost less than 2,000 RMB. Because she was treated away from her place of residence or work and her insurance only covered hospital stays, she had been paying out of pocket for medications. She was not worried about this or about her considerable travel expenses. Every three to four months, she flew back to the east coast specifically to see the doctor, which cost several thousand RMB per journey (TB Interview 27).

Each of these patients was part of China's emerging middle class, which had a growing appetite for goods and services, including healthcare. Like the student studying in Canada, each of these patients traveled regularly. With the exception of the hotel manager's lung cavity (which his first doctor believed might be cancer), the severity of their illnesses did not require money for expensive care, since they had TB strains that were responsive to first-line drugs, yet each chose to travel. Traveling to receive care was an extension of their lifestyle. While the work-unit system was in place, none of these individuals would have had much choice regarding where they received health care. Moreover, opportunities for the accumulation of wealth to enable health-care choice would not have been available if not for the decline of the state-owned sector. Thus, winners in the game of economic change also had the most access to health care and sometimes the best health outcomes.

(Still) Privileged access: State sector employees and retirees

Some of the TB patients I interviewed saw almost no change in their health insurance coverage. Feng Jianping, a 46-year-old man who worked for 26 years in a state-owned steel factory, learned that he had TB during his factory's annual checkup in May 2010. When I interviewed him in December 2010, he had already taken TB medication for about six months. He was worried that his condition had not improved much during this time, and he had recently developed insomnia. Feng was concerned about his own health and about being around for his daughter, who was an international finance major at Shanghai University and hoped to study in America. Something Feng did not need to worry about was health insurance. He had no changes to his out-of-pocket expenses during his 26 years of work. He did not need money when he saw a doctor. Fees were covered by the central and municipal governments (TB Interview 1).

Similarly, individuals who worked for prominent universities still received excellent coverage. He Yi, a 65-year-old retired university professor, discovered he had tuberculosis when he was being treated for another chronic disease at the school's hospital. He was originally from the countryside and brought a thorough written assessment of his own health to his checkup. He was also eager to discuss his health experience with me. His health background included a case of schistosomiasis in 1965, when he was a freshman in college; the disease was discovered through inspection of feces when doctors from the Municipal People's Hospital went to his home. This retired professor also had TB back in the 1980s, but at that time he had such a mild case that he did not take medicine. During his most recent illness, he took medication for one year, which was well covered by insurance (TB Interview 30).

A third respondent, Liu Ying, was a 65-year-old retired office worker from a state-owned commercial enterprise. His work unit had 100 workers and a clinic where they could receive care for common illnesses and injuries. Liu started working there in the 1970s and worked eight-hour days until he retired in 2006.

About a year after he retired, he discovered that he had bone TB. His recovery from the disease was slow. When I spoke to him, he had been in treatment for more than three years. His treatment included two operations and several courses of TB antibiotics. Despite the fact that his illness was complicated and costly, he received reimbursement for 80–90 percent of costs. His son, who was present during the interview, was quick to point out how much better the health insurance of retirees from SOEs was than the insurance of their offspring in today's workforce (TB Interview 9).

Both the steel worker and the retired university professor still received complete coverage for the health expenses they incurred, just as they would have if the work-unit system were still in place. In fact, both of their work units remained fully intact. In Shanghai, it is typical for employees and retirees from privileged SOEs not to have to pay for care. When discussing care more widely, two neighbors in my housing complex who retired from Shanghai Number One Iron and Steel Plant confirmed that their health coverage remained strong. Likewise, among the TB patients I interviewed, Liu Ying, who retired from a successful commercial SOE, also had relatively good coverage. Liu Ying had some out-of-pocket expenses during his three-year treatment regimen, but the health insurance benefits the state provided this retiree were still better than those his son received.

Chapters 4 and 5 demonstrated that even at the height of the work-unit system, not all health-care access was equal. Employees of key state-owned enterprises had better access to tertiary facilities than did employees of collective and workshop enterprises. Rural residents had access to urban tertiary facilities only through referral. In the two decades between 1990 and 2010, inequality of access increased greatly, both within and between sectors. While the number of individuals employed in state-owned enterprises has declined, individuals lucky enough to be employed there were still relatively well covered compared to workers in private enterprises. That state-owned enterprises would continue to provide above-average insurance coverage is not surprising given the government investment in 2000 of 116.8 billion RMB in health insurance for workers in state-owned enterprises, government administration, and public service. However, only 70 million workers, or about 6 percent of China's population, were covered under these schemes (S. Wang 2004). Given that the investment per worker was 1,670 RMB, those who were covered could access the best care available. Unfortunately, the vast majority of the Chinese population, including almost all rural residents and migrant workers, were left out.

While state-owned enterprise employees still enjoyed relative privilege with respect to health insurance and the amount it would cover per illness, one of my respondents who worked in an SOE partially dispelled assumptions about work-unit privilege. This 44-year-old woman worked in a state-owned textile factory in Changzhou that manufactures blue jeans. Much of the structure of health care at her factory remined in place—her factory had a clinic for minor illnesses, provided health checks every two years, and contributed to the cost of her health insurance, which covered three-quarters of expenses per illness—but production expectations had changed, as the factory was now in competition with private enterprises. As a result, workers felt more pressure to meet production targets. This worker did not have a fixed schedule. She had to work all three shifts—morning, evening, and overnight—which affected her sleep and her body's resistance to disease. Sometimes she works seven days a week. When they are busy, she might have one day off every three weeks. If she needs to rest for a day, the factory docks her pay (TB Interview 38). In some ways, her schedule resembled that of textile workers in the Republican era, described in Chapter 2. This worker's experience represents another way workers are now vulnerable: some now have to work longer hours than was permitted under the work-unit system. Exhausting work conditions was a theme in some of my other interview subjects, including the upwardly mobile young professionals, who will be discussed below.

Some access: Laid-off workers and private enterprise employees

The private enterprise employees I interviewed had considerably more variation in terms of what is included in their health plans. One laid-off worker I interviewed who had been able to secure reemployment actually had better health insurance than the commercial worker I interviewed above. Zhao Cheng was a 52-year-old worker from Shanghai's Jiading District. In 1977, at the age of 19, he began working in a state-owned medicine factory with more than 3,000 workers. Since being laid off in 1997, Zhao has worked for a private, Japanese-owned towel factory. The SOE for which he previously worked had an attached hospital. He was eager to emphasize that treatment at the hospital was free: "No need for money! Everything was provided by the government" (TB Interview 33). The hospital arranged for more difficult cases to go elsewhere.

The private factory for which he worked at the time of the interview actually paid a good amount of attention to the health of its employees. Zhao's current workplace invited the CDC to give its workers checkups every year, but his disease was not actually discovered that way. Instead, it was discovered in March 2010, during a follow-up on a case of pneumonia he had in June and July 2009. When he had pneumonia, he stayed in the Jiading Central Hospital for more than 10 days; the bill was more than 6,000 RMB, but his out-of-pocket expense was only 400 RMB. Municipal insurance covered the rest. When he had tuberculosis, he stayed in a municipal-level hospital for 11 days and took medicine for a year. When I interviewed him in February 2011, he was preparing to stop the medicine and said this "felt liberating." He said he would have another CT scan in three months to make sure the disease was not recurring. He said he did not remember the precise amount he spent, but he could confirm that he was reimbursed at a similar rate as he had been when he had pneumonia.

While this worker was relatively pleased with the health insurance coverage he received, another worker I spoke to was more frustrated with the lack of clarity in today's coverage. Yang Xuegong was a 45-year-old Shanghai native whose mother was a general practitioner. He previously worked for a state-owned textile factory with 1,000 workers. Before that company broke up, he sought employment in another private factory. Yang's first factory did a good job of health promotion: it had both loudspeaker announcements about health and announcements posted in the cafeteria. It also provided annual checkups at the Yangpu Central Hospital. His mother is a doctor, so he talks to her right away if he has any illness symptoms. He discovered he had TB because he was extremely tired at work; he then had a bone protrusion characteristic of the type of extrapulmonary TB he had contracted. He had two operations and rested for seven months, from March to October 2009, before beginning work again. When I spoke to him, he was finishing an 18-month course of TB medicine that he had started in May 2009. While he was pleased to complete treatment, he was concerned about reimbursement (TB Interview 8). He had spent 100,000 RMB (US$15,000) out of pocket and had no idea how much of it would be reimbursed. He explained that the current basic health insurance system was not fully in place when he was diagnosed. He expressed nostalgia for the work-unit system under which health coverage had been worry free. Because of his upbringing in a family with a doctor, this patient was knowledgeable about health issues. He paid attention to illness signs and remained abreast of changes to the health system; however, he found the municipal system to be complicated, particularly regarding what can and cannot be reimbursed.

Zhao and Yang were both textile workers and Shanghai natives. Both had worked for state-owned factories that closed in the 1990s, and both were able to secure reemployment in private enterprises, which provided different health benefits. Zhao's workplace provided private insurance, and he was reimbursed for all but 7 percent of his expenses. By contrast, Yang was dealing with higher illness-related expenses and was relying exclusively on the municipal health insurance. Given that he had extrapulmonary TB, Yang's illness was not covered under Shanghai's TB program. There was a fairly good chance that some of his considerable expenses would be covered by the municipal insurance program. The amount he spent exceeded the minimum expense at which pooled funds began to cover expenses, and they did not exceed the maximum. In 2009, Shanghai's average annual per capita GDP was around US$10,000. This meant municipal funds kicked in when US$1,000 was spent for an illness. Pooled funds could no longer be used after expenses exceeded around US$40,000. When he finally sought reimbursement in 2011, municipal insurance would have covered part of his expenses, but at the time of our interview, he could only guess at the amount.

Limited access: Upwardly mobile young professionals

Among some of the younger patients, compromised health due to desire to get ahead was a common theme. Because the frenetic work schedule under the emerging capitalist system had compromised their health, several of my respondents opted to reprioritize their health by taking considerable time off work to recover from their illness. These cases demonstrate patients' commitment to getting well, even if it meant sacrificing part of their family's income or savings, as well as their perception of their own social integration. For instance, several of my respondents took at least six months off work to take care of their health, sometimes because they had extrapulmonary or drug-resistant tuberculosis, which required a complicated regimen of second- or third-line tuberculosis drugs, some of which produced uncomfortable side effects. These patients felt a responsibility to rest, despite the social and financial cost.

Among my youngest interviewees, a 24-year-old recent college graduate attributed his illness to working very long hours in the financial sector. He was a Shanghai native and had graduated from Shanghai University in 2009, approximately one year prior to the discovery of his TB. He started coughing in spring 2010 and went to the hospital after about three months. Since his case was relatively mild, he did not initially take medicine; however, when the condition of his lungs did not improve in the months immediately following the diagnosis, he chose to take medicine and time off from work to recover (TB Interview 26). Had he continued working, he would have had medical insurance. Nonetheless, he was not worried about the cost of medicine and hospital outpatient fees, which were only around 1,000 RMB. His concerns were social: he believed that "100 percent of people show discrimination against TB patients." He worried about whether people would judge him when he tried to go back to work. While he feared discrimination from societal members who do not understand TB, he had made friends through an online chat group with other TB patients, including another of my respondents, which partially mitigated his worry about social integration.

The 24-year-old financial worker's new friends included an opinionated 27-year-old patient from Wenzhou, who felt similar social pressure as a result of her disease. She had gone to college in Shanghai and worked for 2.5 years in the government sector after college. She had a neighbor who died from TB at a young age, which compelled her to take a 2-year leave of absence to recover from

Dismantling of the Work-Unit System and Challenges to Tuberculosis Control 171

her multidrug-resistant TB. Although she did not feel financially compromised by her illness, this patient also expressed social concerns centered around discrimination: "I've never discriminated against anyone—why do they discriminate against me?" (TB Interview 4). Both of these young patients sought out social connections through new media when they felt the scorn of society.

Despite not having to spend time in a sanatorium, some patients chose to spend time in the hospital. In some cases, this was a financial decision, as insurance would only (partially) pay for hospitalization, not outpatient treatment, given the paltry coverage that was initially provided after health reforms intensified in 2009 (TB Interviews 24, 27, and 30). In other cases, patients spent time in the hospital despite the fact that it was not covered by their insurance. For example, a 31-year-old doctor took a long and hopeful view of her illness: she rested for six months, including a month in the hospital. Because she had been working for only a few years, she quickly exhausted the funds in her health spending account, so she spent approximately 20,000 RMB (US$3,000) out of pocket. She was glad she did so: she regained her health and said that she became a better doctor as a result of the experience (TB Interview 16). Patients who chose hospitalization were committed to getting well, even if it meant time away from their families and considerable expense.

Some younger patients worried about whether having the disease would decimate their savings, affecting future life chances. A 21-year-old university student, whose parents were both teachers, had recurring TB. She was from Anhui Province and was studying in Nanjing, but she stated that the insurance provided to university students in Jiangsu was not very comprehensive. She originally had TB four years ago, and her TB had returned 15 months prior to the interview. She coughed for 2 months and was then hospitalized near her home for two weeks. Eventually, she stayed in the Nanjing Chest Hospital for 70 days. Throughout her treatment, she also paid 500–600 RMB per month for medications. All expenses were paid entirely out of pocket. She lamented that the 190,000 RMB she had spent to control her recurring illness was money she might have used to purchase a home (TB Interview 35).

Each of these four respondents was young, college educated, and upwardly mobile, yet each caught TB. Each of them took their sick role seriously and chose to take considerable time off to recover. While the young doctor was able to see a wider lesson from her illness, the others worried about their social mobility. In a society where people have witnessed growing wealth and inequality, TB patients worry about the precariousness of their social position. Buying a home is a particular concern of patients in the post-work-unit era because housing is no longer provided. Moreover, newly wealthy Chinese have invested in real estate, which has driven up prices. This places persons in the difficult position of choosing health over future wealth.

Least access: Migrants

Workers in private enterprises had more confidence in the health system than did the migrants, who amplified some of the themes I had heard from the upwardly mobile young professionals. Zhang Guozheng was a 59-year-old patient with a talkative wife. Both Zhang's background and his illness were somewhat complicated. Zhang was a party member and had been a human resources leader in several stores in Changsha. He was originally laid off at the age of 47. While he found other jobs, his wife had not worked for 15 years. In 2009, he decided to retire, and the couple moved to the wife's ancestral home in Shanghai (TB Interview 13).

He had been coughing, but obtaining a proper diagnosis shortly after he arrived in Shanghai proved problematic. He went to four different hospitals and spent 2,000 RMB before finding his current doctor. At the time of our interview, he had already been in treatment for more than 18 months, battling TB infection of four different organs. His family had spent 70,000–80,000 RMB (over US$10,000) with receipts, but also had some expenses without receipts. Given their status as recent migrants to Shanghai, they were not sure whether any of this money would be reimbursed. Their son used the money with which he intended to buy a house to pay for his father's treatment, which raised questions of how the financial burden from a father's diagnoses would affect the next generation's upward mobility.

Another migrant who had not worked under the work-unit system was a 29-year-old man from Harbin named Ai Jiong. When I interviewed him, Ai and his family had been in Shanghai for 10 years, where they had a machine rental shop. He originally had TB when he was 7 years old. He started coughing again in 2005 and self-medicated with anti-inflammatories and Chinese medicine. Ai did not think much of the cough; when it was severe, he simply took more over-the-counter medicine. When his chest started hurting, he realized it might be TB, saw a doctor, and took medicine for eight months from late spring 2006 to early 2007. During this time, his health deteriorated, and it became clear that he had contracted a drug-resistant strain. At the time of our interview in early 2011, he had been taking second- and third-line TB drugs to combat extremely drug-resistant TB for 4 years. Throughout his treatment, all expenses associated with his illness have been out of pocket, including 130,000 RMB (US$20,000) on medicine and three hospital stays totaling more than 70,000 RMB (more than US$10,000) (TB Interview 29).

Certainly, neither of these migrants' experience represented the typical TB patient in Shanghai, or in China more generally. Both experienced diagnosis delays and required longer, more costly treatment than most of the patients I interviewed. Neither had many expenses that were covered under DOTS or

Dismantling of the Work-Unit System and Challenges to Tuberculosis Control   173

the municipal insurance scheme. Ai Jiong and his family had already lived in Shanghai for more than four years when he started coughing, but neither the municipal insurance scheme nor DOTS covered any of his care. Long-term migrants were not covered under the municipal insurance scheme until 2008, and this was one of the factors involved in his choice to delay seeking care. The XDR strain of TB he contracted required second- and third-line drugs; however, when he was diagnosed, DOTS covered only a standard, six-month course of first-line drugs. Although all districts in Shanghai covered the second- and third-line drugs at the time of our interviews, benefits could be extended retroactively.

Individuals who choose to migrate are generally younger, healthier, and slightly more affluent than other individuals in their sending areas; however, in receiving areas, several possible factors contribute to poorer health. First, migrants often live and work in poorer conditions than do permanent residents. Gone is the day that work units provided housing and limited the hours workers were permitted to be on the job. While the housing provided by work units was often overcrowded and families did not always have their own kitchen or bathroom, families did have permanent walls and a bed. In urban China today, among the employment sectors notorious for putting migrants' health at risk are the construction sector and entertainment industry. Construction workers often live in makeshift dwellings on the perimeter of construction sites, where they live in bunks, with more than six persons per room (Swider 2015). Likewise, the staff in beauty and massage parlors that operate late at night might become vulnerable, because of lack of sleep. They have been known to sleep on the couches or chairs in the entryway of these establishments during the day or on massage tables that are not in use.[3] Consequently, the distal causes of disease transmission that were once mitigated by housing and other benefits supplied by the work-unit system have become an issue once again.

Additionally, migrants are more mobile and consequently, may have less frequent contact with the health system than do permanent residents. As noted above, migrants were excluded from Shanghai's TB control program until 2003 and its basic urban insurance system until 2008. This means that they had to pay out of pocket at the time services were rendered at health facilities. Prior to 2003, migrants throughout China had to return to their official residence to receive TB treatment. Even after coverage expanded in 2003 and 2008, migrants did not interact with the health-care system at the grassroots level, as their parents once did. As demonstrated in Chapters 4 and 5, workplace doctors, including barefoot

---

3. I accidentally awakened the "beauticians" when I visited their shop in the middle of the day during research in 2009. A Chinese friend pointed out that they likely also provided sexual services. This sort of establishment was the setting for Sandra Hyde's ethnographic research on prostitution in Yunnan's border region, Shishuangbanna.

doctors in the countryside, understood the living and working conditions of the people they served. Since the decline of these programs, barriers between elite medical providers and their patients have been raised once again. Today's doctors are less familiar with the conditions of the patients they serve and, consequently, are less able to advocate for them.

It should be noted that my sampling method allowed me to interview only TB patients, not those who forego care, yet I still found considerable variation in level of care, as well as in disease complexity. All respondents viewed their own health as important enough to make the financial sacrifice, paying out of pocket, as necessary. Each of the interviewees stated that they were able to meet the considerable cost associated with their illness, which totaled as much as US$30,000. Their ability to meet these expenses raises questions about those who are not able to pay. If these individuals or their relatives had not had the savings necessary to cover their costs, would they have had to forego treatment? In a patchwork system where neither the municipal insurance program nor the DOTS program met many of the expenses incurred by TB patients, especially by migrants, this was a big concern.

To summarize, the data from the interviews with TB patients indicated that the decline of the work-unit system resulted in a spectrum of coverage. Some individuals were able to become wealthy, and consequently, they were not concerned about the cost of care. In the second tier, employees and retirees in the state-owned university system and other privileged state-owned industries, such as steel factories, had relatively strong access, though working conditions had declined for some. As demonstrated, health insurance coverage for workers in private enterprises and for young individuals starting their careers varied. For migrants, coverage was often not very good and might involve diagnosis delays or treatment interruptions, leading to a more complicated, lengthy, and costly care regimen. Age was also a crucial variable in my analysis. Older patients tended to nostalgically focus on the past—emphasizing how decline of the social security system led to rising out-of-pocket costs. By contrast, younger patients worried about how the disease provided a challenge to social integration, as well as their prospects for the future.

Shanghai saw fundamental structural change, and these changes influenced patients' experience. In the first decade of the twenty-first century, TB was both an opportunistic and an anachronistic disease—remaining stubbornly part of Chinese society, despite phenomenal economic growth. Shanghai currently has some of China's most advanced health facilities, and these facilities are open to anyone who can pay, but health insurance coverage in the postsocialist era was incomplete. Persons who were left behind during China's rise as a global economic powerhouse found themselves most vulnerable to disease, with the fewest resources for treatment. Further consideration of these individuals' plight is vitally important during an era of renewed concern about pandemics and how to prevent their spread.

* * *

During my 2008–2012 fieldwork, Shanghai saw reinvigoration of TB educational campaigns, with district CDCs largely leading these efforts. Large-screen flash advertisements from the central and district CDCs played in public spaces such as shopping centers, and public service announcements played on closed-circuit televisions on public transportation. District CDCs also distributed seasonal marketing items, such as fans and umbrellas. The Changning CDC provided calendars with TB prevention slogans to children when they visited schools, and the Putuo CDC distributed magnetic bookmarks with the popular Chinese cartoon character Pleasant Goat (喜羊羊) (Providers 30 and 34). Each year, targeted, week-long public education campaigns coincided with International TB Awareness Day on March 24. Local papers printed articles to make the public aware of TB's symptoms, with instructions on where to receive free treatment. In honor of International TB Awareness Day, some universities held lectures and university hospital staff tabled to raise students' and employees' awareness and knowledge of disease (Provider 19). District-level facilities coordinated with university personnel in these efforts. As we saw in the previous chapter, at least one district CDC participated in university efforts by holding contests in which students earn monetary prizes for designing educational campaign materials (Provider 27). In 2011, my host university also held various events, including tabling to raise the TB awareness among students and staff. These programs aimed to bring TB prevention knowledge to schools, as some Republican-era health campaigns aimed to do and district TB prevention and treatment clinics did in workplaces, from the 1950s to 1992.

Conclusions

Fundamental changes occurred in urban China starting in the 1990s. The cradle-to-grave security the work-unit system once offered most urban residents and their families disappeared as permanent employment and workplace benefits were eliminated during the process of privatization of state-owned and collective enterprises. In addition, private enterprises made their debut in Shanghai's industrial and rapidly expanding service sector. Private enterprises offered fewer benefits to their workers than had SOEs and COEs, but Shanghai saw no shortage of individuals willing to take jobs in the private sector. As illustrated above, some of these enterprises have allowed their employees to accumulate wealth, which has given them ample choices about accessing healthcare.

With respect to health insurance, Shanghai's municipal government has stepped up to partially replace lost benefits; however, coverage was not nearly as good as it was when the work-unit system was fully in place. Shanghai's basic health insurance, which was introduced in 1996, helped to defray costs of non-catastrophic illnesses, but the portion of health expenses borne by individual families increased dramatically between 1990 and 2000. Families were responsible for bearing all costs associated with health conditions less than 10 percent of Shanghai's average annual wage with their individual health accounts or their savings. Families were also responsible for all medical expenses beyond four times the average annual wage. As noted above, these expenses affected the poor, laid-off workers, and migrant workers more than they did wealthy individuals. In the realm of TB control, the DOTS program was designed to be universally applied; however, that program is inferior to the TB control provided at the grass-roots level when the work-unit system was fully in place. DOTS has coverage exclusions as well as problems with its case finding and treatment models. Out-of-pocket costs for healthcare rose for both Shanghai residents and migrants, often contributing to delays in care seeking and poorer treatment management. Shanghai was slow to respond to the obstacles faced by both the urban population and its influx of migrants. These problems contributed to TB control challenges starting the mid-1990s and were only partially corrected through reforms in the 2000s. This has been changing, as equity concerns have become more central in the most recent decade.

Conclusion

China is critically important to global health. The 2002–2003 SARS epidemic set off alarm bells for needed change. With the 2004 Revised Law on the Prevention and Control of Infectious Diseases, China began to reprioritize disease control. Most of the data for this book were collected after this law had been in place for only a few years, when health access inequalities were particularly stark. In the 2010s, equity concerns became more central to health reforms. Thus, China has been working to overcome some of the variation in access to TB control around 2010 that this research uncovered. With respect to controlling faster-acting and deadlier respiratory diseases, such as COVID-19, China's commitment remains strong. China was one of the only nations to continue to maintain a zero-COVID policy until December 2022.

Although China's critical role in global health today cannot be denied, scholarship of the past two decades has elevated the importance of the most populous nation in our understanding of colonial health in the early twentieth century, international health and development in the postwar era, and global health since the 1980s. This book has woven an important yarn into the conversation by examining tuberculosis, which was consistently the world's most widespread and deadliest infectious disease, until the onset of COVID-19. In closing, we return to some of the past's most important lessons for the present.

Situating Shanghai's TB Control within International Health, Development, and Global Health

Disease remains a potential threat to the nation and national reputation on the international stage. This is as true today, with the rise of COVID-19, as it was in the first half of the twentieth century, when nation after nation began to grapple with tuberculosis. Throughout the twentieth century, disease tied closely to economic modernization, with those living in poorer conditions and without access to modern sanitation, nutrition, or health care most susceptible. This was true in the colonial era, the era of socialist modernization, and the era of market socialism. This book has illustrated that even though the term "global health" did not come into vogue until the 1980s, public health officials in China were influenced by public health movements happening on an international and global scale, even in the early twentieth century when TB was a global concern.

Given the social disruption that accompanied regime change in the first decades of the twentieth century, the Chinese state was late to begin anti-TB and other public health work, and it did so only in a limited capacity, even in its largest and most economically advanced city. International health was closely tied to colonial enterprises, including in China. This is particularly evident looking at the Shanghai Municipal Council Health Department's approach to health. As illustrated in Chapter 1, the Municipal Health Department was originally only concerned with the health of Chinese citizens only insofar as it affected the health of foreign citizens. As the years progressed, the short sightedness of this vision became clear, and the SMC began to take a more pressing interest in Chinese residents. War slowed down these changes in 1915–1919, and the SMC never went so far as to address underlying social conditions. Yet with changes to leadership in both the SMC Health Department and the Chinese GMD government, state actors began to pay more attention to more distal causes of disease.

The social determinants of health came into focus in the interwar years, and with this focus came a belief that medicine should be a social endeavor. Organizations dedicated to promoting social medicine on a global stage, such as the Rockefeller Foundation and the League of Nations Health Organization, entered China with gusto for the work to be done (Birn 2009; Borowy 2009; Brazelton 2020, 2021; Zhou 2020). Under the GMD government, China was motivated to control disease, to overcome the label of the "sick man of Asia" and strengthen the nation. As the leading infectious disease in China, TB was part of this focus; however, as was the case in 1915–1919, war interrupted some of these efforts and contributed to increased TB, particularly in overcrowded cities. The Shanghai Anti-Tuberculosis Association arose to combat this challenge, and TB control work of the final GMD years and Mao era built upon the foundation laid during the war.

After the Second World War, international health improvements became tied closely to the international development project. States were important actors attempting to demonstrate the superiority of their economic model and its accompanying institutions through widespread gains in health. Starting in the 1950s, the Chinese state developed a way to bring new scientific advances to its citizens, thus demonstrating the strength of socialist modernization. Scientization was central to these plans, and a growing body of work has demonstrated how science became a tool for consolidating social control and creating a new reality during the Mao era (Gross 2016; Schmalzer 2016; Ghosh 2020). Chinese officials were quick to construct a narrative that improving quality of life and life

Conclusion   179

expectancy demonstrated the superiority of the socialist model. As Chapters 3–4 illustrate, through the ubiquitous work-unit system, China succeeded in delivering housing, food, health insurance, and other social welfare benefits. Thus, quality of life and life expectancy improved for many urban workers in Shanghai. However, the health gains were not evenly felt, either within Shanghai or beyond.

The gradations and unevenness felt during the Mao era were exacerbated in by post-1980s neoliberalism and globalization. In 1978, China had already begun to turn away from the socialist economic model. In urban areas, the work-unit system remained largely in place until the 1990s; however, as the new economic model found its way into the Chinese countryside, the commune and its associated health system underwent dramatic transformation. Chapter 5 demonstrated that Shanghai's rural counties saw improvements to the credentialing of village doctors and expansion of infrastructure, but Shanghai was an anomalous case. Generally, China's turn away from primary health care in rural areas paralleled that of the world. Worldwide, the new era of "global health" actually prioritized economic interests over health. This was the same time frame during which China was normalizing relations with much of the world, leading to an exponential expansion in global interactions, including trade.

In a new era of globalization and interconnection, which emerged in the 1980s, newly emerging and reemerging diseases, like SARS, bird flu, COVID-19, and MDR-TB, have capitalized on persistent inequality. Both the Chinese government and international scholars have linked emerging epidemics to capitalist excess. For example, Gewirtz points out that China calls AIDS "loving capitalism disease," stemming from a belief that "AIDS represented the underside of globalized, capitalistic modernity," which could be avoided by embracing virtuous socialist living and avoiding "decadent" lifestyles (Gewirtz 2020: 253). This logic might be seen as a continuation of the culture of disease control established in the 1950s that has continued to be employed to control recent global pandemics. While Gerwitz's argument focuses on state attention to individual behaviors, other scholars have warned against many other negative externalities of capitalism. As Mike Davis cautions in his recently updated volume on bird flu, "Multinational capital has been the driver of disease evolution through the burning or logging out of tropical forest, the proliferation of factory farming, the explosive growth of slums and concomitantly of 'informal employment,' and the failure of the pharmaceutical industry to find profit in mass producing lifeline antivirals, new-generation antibiotics, and universal vaccines" (Davis 2022: 17). Likewise, Li Zhang (2021) identifies global capitalism as the driving force behind COVID-19. Indeed, institutions matter for preventing disease from exploiting systemic inequalities.

Continuity and Change in Welfare Provision and Inequality

As models of international health shifted in the mid-twentieth century, China often saw only minor shifts with respect to state attention and commitment to health and welfare provisions, organizational forms, and the persistence of inequality. As the leader of the first Chinese state in the "modern era," the GMD envisioned improving citizens' health but faced challenges to doing so. The New Life Movement focused on creating healthier citizens, yet the movement was largely driven by the upper classes and often excluded and stigmatized the lower classes. During the National Health Reconstruction there was some follow-through with respect to welfare provision. For example, privileged heavy industries, such as munitions, already saw state commitment to social protections. Thus, there was some continuity in the state's desire to provide necessities under different governments—GMD, Maoist, and Reform—but the follow-through mechanism changed substantially.

What was lacking under the GMD government was a grassroots mechanism of reaching, motivating, and controlling individual members of the population. This volume has demonstrated that the work unit became the institution for inculcating, enculturating, and cajoling the masses with respect to health. This pervasive urban organizational form persisted into the 1990s, when dramatic institutional change occurred. Yet the effects of such a pervasive system were still felt with respect to who had access to care and the type of care they received well into the twenty-first century.

Even in the Mao era, inequality persisted in several ways. The biggest persistent inequality this book identified is unequal access to quality health care among Shanghai's residents based upon their place of employment and residential status. Workers in privileged industries had access to the best hospitals, while those in less privileged industries had less access. The work-unit system solidified these inequalities for many years, as the system held everyone in place. Moreover, those in rural areas were at a disadvantage, as the residence-permit system provided a barrier to entering urban areas.

Starting in the 1980s, economic reform amplified differential access to medical care. As Chapter 6 demonstrates, a decade into the twenty-first century, the type of care one was able to get depended upon one's workplace. Those with means were able to access high-quality care, while levels of medical debt grew for those whose workplaces did not grant generous welfare contributions. Medical protests increased as the realization of the right to health care became compromised. The public health system saw some recovery after the 2003 SARS epidemic, and the state paid greater attention to providing more equitable care for citizens in the 2010s. While the national government has focused on remedies to health inequalities, this book has not endeavored to examine regional

Conclusion 181

inequalities among provinces, which has led to the prioritization of urban metropolises (Jaros 2019).

China and Global Health: Lessons for the Present

Finding ways to reach the public is critically important for the success of public health interventions, particularly those aimed at controlling respiratory diseases. Reaching members of the population for health interventions is always difficult, regardless of income and education level. Several lessons from TB control in China are relevant to the COVID-19 pandemic elsewhere in the world.

First, high levels of social control can be important for efficiently squelching infectious disease outbreaks. As intrusive as it was, the work-unit system worked well for disease control. Strict, often invasive surveillance allows the state to count and control members of the population. Indeed, authoritarian countries with strict control of their populations are able to implement strict disease control measures today. As COVID outbreaks have occurred, China continued to lock down various geographical areas, sometimes including entire neighborhoods and cities, throughout 2020–2022. Other nations, such as the United States and the United Kingdom took a different approach, prioritizing individual liberty over safety, which initially resulted in more infections and deaths.

The social structure, with work units as central, ubiquitous, privileged members, allowed for several disease-control mechanisms to function efficiently. Among those mechanisms, widespread case finding is important, and some sort of follow-up is equally necessary. Starting after the Japanese Occupation, urban China underwent widespread case finding. As a follow-up to case finding, work units allowed their workers to take time off, so that they could rest and recover from TB. During their convalescence, work unit members were supported. Work units in China often created spaces for sick individuals to isolate. Indeed, isolation of suspected cases remains important and challenging in crowded urban environments, regardless of the disease in question.

In China, work units also met the fundamental need for shelter, which served both a manifest and latent function. Granted, there was unevenness in housing provision, and many urban dwellings remained relatively crowded; however, having stable walls and a roof are preferable to makeshift camps. This improved immunity and reduced chances for transmission. Work-unit housing also provided a latent function with respect to disease control: surveillance. Living and working with people from the same "unit" allowed workers to police behavior on issues as small as fashion choices or as important as infectious disease control. Both historically and in the present day, neighborhood committees have also served as local-level state actors who step in to provide services or surveillance as necessary.

When it comes to treatment, improving health-care access is key. In China under the work-unit system, health care was provided for work unit members. Granted, quality of care varied between the city and countryside, as well as among work units, and the system never covered all urban residents; however, high levels of coverage prevented difficult economic decisions about which bills to pay. Now China struggles to actualize the right to health care, but it maintains a strong commitment to treating TB and to isolating and treating sufferers of newly emerging diseases. This state commitment continued into the COVID-19 pandemic. These are important lessons for the twenty-first century, when better institutions are needed to protect the poorest among us to improve the safety for all.

Appendix: Tuberculosis Patient Interviewees

Number	Age	Sex	Residence	Occupation / employment situation	Social class
1	46	M	Shanghai	Worker, employed for 26 years in a state-owned steel factory.	Working
2	33	M	Zhejiang, came to Shanghai only for treatment	Worker in the food and beverage industry.	Working
3	52	M	Taizhou, Zhejiang, came to only Shanghai for treatment	Owner of a small factory that makes towels.	Self-employed
4	33	F	Shanghai	Stable employment in water management for 7.5 years, since graduate school.	Middle
5	27	F	Wenzhou, Zhejiang, came to Shanghai only for treatment	(Attended university in Shanghai). Currently on 2-year sick leave from a government office in Wenzhou.	Middle
6	22	F	Northern Jiangsu province, came to Shanghai only for treatment	Just graduated from university where she was a computer science major.	Middle
7	28	F	Originally from Shanghai, but recently spent 2–3 months in Zhangzhou, Henan	Her husband's family is in the real estate business, where she has been working for 5–6 years since marriage.	Middle
8	45	M	Shanghai	Worked for an SOE with 1,000 workers. Before that company broke up, he already sought employment elsewhere.	Working

Number	Age	Sex	Residence	Occupation / employment situation	Social class
9	65	M	Zhenzhou, came to Shanghai only for treatment	Office worker in a commerce SOE. Started work in the 1970s; retired 4–5 years ago.	Working
10	38	F	Anhui Province, came to Shanghai only for treatment	Not currently working (because her husband does not want her to, given her XDR diagnosis). Was a tour guide and worked in a store before getting married in 2005.	Working
11	36	F	Anhui countryside (near Hefei), came to Shanghai only for treatment	Started doing manual labor at the age of 17. Currently a homemaker with two children (ages 13 and 7).	Working poor
12	28	F	From Hangzhou, came to Shanghai only for treatment	Works in a family-owned shop.	Self-employed
13	59	M	Changsha, but recently moved to Shanghai, his wife's ancestral home	Worked in human resources in several stores but retired in 2009. Originally laid off at 47 years old. Wife hasn't had salary for 15 years.	Working
14	27	M	Taizhou, Zhejiang, came to Shanghai only for treatment	From an entrepreneurial family. They used to sell shoes, but have been selling pants for 2 years.	Self-employed
15	66	F	Shanghai	Worked as a hospital cashier for 34 years starting in 1967. Retired 11 years ago.	Middle
16	31	F	Shanghai	Doctor of Western medicine; came to Shanghai for residency and has been working for 6 years.	Middle
17	33	F	Taizhou, Zhejiang, came to Shanghai only for treatment	Part-time cab driver—worked ages 16–26; stopped working after she got married.	Working
18	25	F	Suzhou (new countryside), came to Shanghai only for treatment	Secretary at an electric company.	Working

Appendix

Number	Age	Sex	Residence	Occupation / employment situation	Social class
19	28	M	Shanghai	IT sector, was a computer science major in college.	Middle
20	38	F	Suzhou, came to Shanghai only for treatment	Garment worker; husband is a day laborer.	Working
21	31	F	Shanghai	Currently working as an engineer in a private company. Previously worked as a teacher.	Middle
22	20	F	Hefei, came to Shanghai only for treatment	Student at a university in Canada.	Upper Middle
23	24	F	From Chongqing, but has resided in Shanghai for 5 years	She does not work. She stays at home and is supported by her boyfriend.	Working
24	23	F	From Anhui, but has resided in Shanghai for 4 years	Previously worked in Zhejiang. Has been resting for 2–3 years since giving birth.	Migrant workers
25	69	M	Shanghai	Attended university in China's west. Worked in the Shanghai suburbs; now retired.	Middle
26	24	M	Shanghai	Financial sector following graduation from Shanghai University in 2009.	Middle
27	38	F	Wenzhou, Zhejiang, came to Shanghai only for treatment	Successful businesswoman. Got her start at age 15 at a beauty parlor in Shandong, where she worked for 8 years. Currently sells Dell computers in Sichuan.	Self-employed
28	37	F	Guilin, came to Shanghai only for treatment	Government worker.	Middle
29	29	M	From Heilongjiang, but has resided in Shanghai for 10 years	His family sells machinery.	Self-employed

Number	Age	Sex	Residence	Occupation / employment situation	Social class
30	65	M	Shanghai (originally from the countryside)	Retired university professor.	Middle
31	22	M	Shanghai	Sanitation inspector.	Working
32	54	M	Ningbo, came to Shanghai only for treatment	Management in private (armed) security company for more than 10 years. Started working at age 24; used to be a professor.	Middle
33	52	M	Shanghai (Jiading District)	Textile worker; began working in 1977 at age 19. He used to work for an SOE with more than 3,000 workers. Since being laid off in 1997, he works for a Japanese private towel factory.	Working
34	29	F	From Harbin, has been in Shanghai for 5 years	Works with computers for a private Hong Kong company at a call center answering calls mostly from within China.	Middle
35	21	F	Huangshan in Anhui, came to Shanghai only for treatment	Studying at a university in Nanjing. Both of her parents are teachers.	Middle
36	34	M	Yuyao, Zhejiang Province, came to Shanghai only for treatment	Has held several jobs in foreign trade for 14 years.	Middle
37	31	F	Hangzhou, came to Shanghai only for treatment	Nurse, working for 10 years.	Middle
38	44	F	Changzhou, came to Shanghai only for treatment	Textile worker in a state-owned jeans factory with 2,000-plus workers for 22 years.	Working
39	21	M	Shanghai (Fengxian District)	Undergraduate in communication engineering (in Hunan Province) but wants to be a fashion designer.	Middle

Number	Age	Sex	Residence	Occupation / employment situation	Social class
40	23	M	Shanghai	Goes to Shanghai University, internship is in Jiading District, where he had planned to work after graduation.	Middle
41	48	F	Shanghai (Pudong District)	Worked in a factory until the first time she had TB in 1994.	Working
42	58	F	Gansu province, came to Shanghai only for treatment	Doesn't really work; her husband is a day laborer.	Working poor
43	26	F	Fujian, came to Shanghai only for treatment	College educated, has worked in sales for 4–5 years, 8 hours per day, 5.5 days per week.	Middle
44	36	M	Hohot, Inner Mongolia. Previously lived in Shanghai and returned for treatment	Works as a manager for a hotel group. Started working in Guangzhou when he graduated from high school in 1994. Has also lived in Beijing, Shanghai, and Shandong.	Middle; Managerial
45	30	M	From Shizhou in Zhejiang, came to Shanghai only for treatment	Has worked for 10 years.	Working

References

Abu-Lughod, Janet. 1989. *Before European Hegemony: The World System A.D. 1250–1350.* New York: Oxford University Press.

Alexander, Peter and Anita Chan. 2004. "Does China Have an Apartheid Pass System?" *Journal of Ethnic and Migration Studies* 30(4): 609–29.

Altman, Lawrence K. 2008. "Drug-Resistant TB Rates Soar in Former Soviet Regions." *New York Times*, February 27.

Anagnost, Ann S. 2007. "Strange Circulations: The Blood Economy in Rural China." *Economy and Society* 35(4): 509–29.

Anderson, Warwick. 1995. "Excremental Colonialism: Public Health and the Poetics of Pollution." *Critical Inquiry* 21(3): 640–69.

Andreas, Joel. 2012. "Industrial Restructuring and Class Transformation in China." Pp. 102–23 in *China's Peasants and Workers: Changing Class Identities*, edited by B. Carrillo and D. Goodman. Northampton, MA: Edward Elgar.

Andrews, Bridie. 1997. "Tuberculosis and the Assimilation of Germ Theory in China, 1885–1937." *Journal of the History of Medicine and Allied Sciences* 52(1): 114–57.

Andrews, Bridie. 2011. "In Republican China, Public Health by Whom, for Whom?" Pp. 177–94 in *Science, Public Health and the State in Modern Asia*, edited by L. Bu, D. Stapleton, and K. C. Yip. New York: Routledge.

Andrews, Bridie. 2014. *The Making of Modern Chinese Medicine, 1850–1960.* Honolulu: University of Hawai'i Press.

Andrews, Bridie. 2015. "Ding Fubao and the Morals of Medical Modernization." *East Asian Science, Technology, and Medicine* 42 (special issue): 7–38.

Arnold, David. 1991. *Colonizing the Body: State Medicine and Epidemic Disease in Nineteenth-Century India.* Berkeley: University of California Press.

Ash, Robert. 1981. "The Quest for Food Self-Sufficiency." Pp. 188–221 in *Shanghai: Revolution and Development in an Asian Metropolis*, edited by C. Howe. Cambridge: Cambridge University Press.

Barnes, David S. 1995. *The Making of a Social Disease: Tuberculosis in Nineteenth Century France.* Berkeley: University of California Press.

Barnes, Nicole Elizabeth. 2018. *Intimate Communities: Wartime Healthcare and the Birth of Modern China, 1937–1945.* Berkeley: University of California Press.

Barnes, Nicole Elizabeth. 2022. "Health and State Making: The Expansion of State Health Services during the War of Resistance against Japan (1937–45)." *Twentieth-Century China* 47(1): 60–70.

References

Barnes, Nicole Elizabeth, and John Watt. 2014. "The Influence of War on China's Modern Health Systems." Pp. 227–43 in *Medical Transitions in Twentieth-Century China*, edited by B. Andrews and M. B. Bullock. Bloomington: University of Indiana Press.

Basilico, Matthew, Jonathan Weigel, Anjali Motgi, Jacob Bor, and Salmaan Keshavjee. 2013. "Health for All? Competing Theories and Geopolitics." Pp. 74–110 in *Reimagining Global Health: An Introduction*, edited by P. Farmer, J. Y. Kim, A. Kleinman, and M. Basilico. Berkeley: University of California Press.

Bates, Barbara. 1992. *Bargaining for Life: A Social History of Tuberculosis, 1876–1938*. Philadelphia: University of Pennsylvania Press.

Baum, Emily. 2018. *The Invention of Madness: State, Society, and the Insane in Modern China*. Chicago: University of Chicago Press.

Beaubien, Jason. 2013. "Love in the Time of TB: A Young Family Fights an Ancient Foe." National Public Radio, *All Things Considered*, June 3, 2013.

Benedict, Carol. 1996. *Bubonic Plague in Nineteenth Century China*. Palo Alto, CA: Stanford University Press.

Bergère, Marie-Claire. 2009. *Shanghai: China's Gateway to Modernization*. Stanford, CA: Stanford University Press.

Bhattacharyya, Onil, Yin Delu, Sabrina T. Wong, and Chen Bowen. 2011. "Evolution of Primary Care in China 1997–2009." *Health Policy* 100: 174–80.

Bian, Morris L. 2005. *The Making of the State Enterprise System in Modern China: The Dynamics of Institutional Change*. Cambridge, MA: Harvard University Press.

Bian, Yanjie. 1994. *Work and Inequality in Urban China*. Albany: State University of New York Press.

Bian, Yanjie, John R. Logan, Hanlong Lu, Yunkang Pan, and Yung Guan. 1997. "Work Units and Housing Reform in Two Chinese Cities." Pp. 223–50 in *Danwei: The Changing Chinese Workplace in Historical and Comparative Perspective*, edited by X. Lü and E. J. Perry. Armonk, NY: M. E. Sharpe.

Birn, Anne-Emanuelle. 2009. "The Stages of International (Global) Health: Histories of Success or Successes of History." *Global Public Health* 4(1): 50–68.

Blumenthal, David and William Hsiao. 2005. "Privatization and Its Discontents: The Evolving Chinese Health Care System." *New England Journal of Medicine* 353: 1165–70.

Borgdorff, Martien W., Katherine Floyd, and Jaap F. Broekmans. 2002. "Interventions to Reduce Tuberculosis Mortality and Transmission in Low- and Middle-Income Countries." *Bulletin of the World Health Organization* 80(3): 217–27.

Borowy, Iris. 2009. *Coming to Terms with World Health: The League of Nations Health Organization, 1921–46*. Frankfurt: Peter Lang.

Bowers, John Z. 1974. "American Private Aid at Its Peak: Peking Union Medical College." Pp. 82–99 in *Medicine and Society in China*, edited by J. Z. Bowers and E. Purcell. New York: Josiah Macy, Jr. Foundation.

Bramall, Chris. 2009. *Chinese Economic Development*. London: Routledge.

Brazelton, Mary Augusta. 2019a. "Coping with Danger in the Air: BCG Vaccination in the Republic of China and International Projects of Postwar Tuberculosis Control, 1930–1949." *Cross-Currents: East Asian History and Culture Review* 30: 35–54.

Brazelton, Mary Augusta. 2019b. *Mass Vaccination: Citizens' Bodies and State Power in Modern China*. Ithaca, NY: Cornell University Press.

Brazelton, Mary Augusta. 2020. "Viral Reflections: Placing China in Global Health Histories." *Journal of Asian Studies* 79(3): 579–88.

Brazelton, Mary Augusta. 2021. "Health for All? Histories of International and Global Health." *History Compass*, e12700. Accessed December 20, 2021 (https://doi.org/10.1111/hic3.12700).

Brook, Timothy. 2005. *Collaboration: Japanese Agents and Local Elites in Wartime China*. Cambridge, MA: Harvard University Press.

Brown, Jeremy. 2012. *City v. Countryside in Mao's China: Negotiating the Divide*. New York: Cambridge University Press.

Brown, Jeremy and Paul Pickowicz. 2012. "The Early Years of the People's Republic of China: An Introduction." Pp. 1–18 in *Dilemmas of Victory*, edited by J. Brown and P. Pickowicz. Cambridge, MA: Harvard University Press.

Brownell, Susan. 1995. *Training the Body for China: Sports in the Moral Order of the People's Republic*. Chicago: University of Chicago Press.

Bryder, Linda. 1988. *Below the Magic Mountain: A Social History of Tuberculosis in Twentieth-Century Britain*. New York: Oxford University Press.

Bu, Liping. 2009. "Public Health and Modernization: The First Campaigns in China, 1915–16." *Social History of Medicine* 22(2): 305–19.

Bu, Liping. 2017. *Public Health and the Modernization of China, 1865–2015*. London: Routledge.

Buck, Daniel. 2012. *Constructing China's Capitalism: Shanghai and the Nexus of Urban-Rural Industries*. New York: Palgrave MacMillan.

Bukhman, Gene. 2001. "Reform and Resistance in Post-Soviet Tuberculosis Control." PhD dissertation, University of Arizona.

Burns, Lawton and Gordon G. Liu. 2017. "China's Healthcare Industry: A System Perspective." Pp. 3–30 in *China's Healthcare System and Reform*, edited by Lawton Robert Burns and Gordon G. Liu. New York: Cambridge University Press.

Cain, Kevin P., Stephen R. Benoit, Carla A. Winston, and William MacKenzie. 2008. "Tuberculosis among Foreign-Born Persons in the United States." *Journal of the American Medical Association* 300(4): 405–12.

Chan, Kam Wing. 2012. "Migration and Development in China: Trends, Geography, and Current Issues." *Migration and Development* 1(20): 187–205.

Chan, Kam Wing and Will Buckingham. 2008. "Is China Abolishing the *Hukou* System?" *China Quarterly* 195: 582–606.

Chang, Jung. 1991. *Wild Swans: Three Daughters of China*. New York: Simon & Schuster.

Chen, Janet Y. 2012. *Guilty of Indigence: The Urban Poor in China, 1900–1953*. Princeton, NJ: Princeton University Press.

Chen, Jing, Lihong Qi, Zhen Xia, Mei Shen, Xin Shen, Jian Mei, Kathryn DeRiemer, and Zheng'an Yuan. 2013. "Which Migrants Default from Tuberculosis Treatment in Shanghai?" *PLoS ONE* 8(11): e81351.

Chen, Lincoln and Ling Chen. 2014. "China's Exceptional Health Transitions: Overcoming the Four Horsemen of the Apocalypse." Pp. 17–31 in *Medical Transitions in*

Twentieth-Century China, edited by B. Andrews and M. B. Bullock. Bloomington: University of Indiana Press.

Chen, Meei-shia. 2001. "The Great Reversal: Transformation of Health Care in the People's Republic of China." Pp. 456–82 in *The Blackwell Companion to Medical Sociology,* edited by W. C. Cockerham. Oxford, U.K.: Blackwell.

Chen Weitang and Sun Gensheng (陈维糖, 孙艮生). 1954. "Introduction to the Medical Situation at Shanghai's Fifth National Cotton Factory Self-Built Sanitarium" (上海国棉五厂自办疗养所务情况介绍). *Shanghai Anti-Tuberculosis* (上海防痨) 4(1): 7–9.

Chen, Xianyi, Fengzeng Zhao, Hongjin Duanmu, Liya Wan, Lixia Wang, Xin Du, and Daniel P. Chin. 2002. "The DOTS Strategy in China: Results and Lessons after Ten Years." *Bulletin of the World Health Organization* 80(2): 430–36.

Chen, Zhiqiang, Guocheng Zhang, Xiangdong Gong, Charles Lin, Xing Gao, Guojun Liang, Xiaoli Yue, Xiangsheng Chen, and Myron S. Cohen. 2007. "Syphilis in China: Results of a National Surveillance Programme." *Lancet* 369 (January 13): 132–38.

Chen, Zhu. 2011. "Healthcare System Reform in China." *World Medical Journal* 59: 8–12.

Child Labor Commission. 1924. "Report of the Child Labor Commission." *Municipal Gazette* 17: 259–70.

China Anti-Tuberculosis Association (CATA中国防痨协会). 1954. "1953 BCG Work Summary Report." *Anti-TB Journal* 《防痨通讯》 7(4): 17–19.

China Anti-Tuberculosis Journal (中国防痨杂志编者), ed. 1965. "Put Medicine and Health Work Emphasis on the Countryside" (一定要把医药卫生工作重点放到农村去). 6(6): 341.

China Medical Association (CMA) TB Study Division (中华医学会结核病学分会). 1997. 中国结核病学科发展史). *History of the Development of the Scientific Study of Tuberculosis in China*. Beijing: Modern China Press.

China Tuberculosis Control Collaboration. 2004. "The Effect of Tuberculosis Control in China." *Lancet* 364 (July 31, 2004): 417–22.

Christensen, Carlo. 1968. "The First Christmas Seal." *Childhood Education* 45(4): 212.

Cockerham, William. 1999. *Health and Social Change in Russia and Eastern Europe*. New York: Routledge.

Cook, Sarah. 1999. "Creating Welfare and Wealth: Entrepreneurship and the Developmental State in Rural China." *IDS Bulletin* 30(4): 60–70.

Core, Rachel. 2014. "Tuberculosis Control in Shanghai: Bringing Health to the Masses, 1928–Present." Pp. 126–45 in *Medical Transitions in Twentieth-Century China*, edited by B. Andrews and M. B. Bullock. Bloomington: University of Indiana Press.

Core, Rachel. 2015. "The Fall and Rise of Tuberculosis: How Institutional Change Affected Health Outcomes in Shanghai, 1927–2013." *Fudan Journal of Humanities and Social Sciences* 9: 65–90.

Core, Rachel. 2019. "Tuberculosis Control, Institutional Change and the Fundamental Causes of Disease in Shanghai: Continuity and Change in Pre- and Post-1949 Shanghai." *American Journal of Chinese Studies* 26(2): 73–89.

Core, Rachel. 2022. "The People's Health: Health Intervention and Delivery in Mao's China, 1949–83, by Xun Zhou." *China Journal* 88: 170–72.

Cui Xiang (催祥). 1966. "Suggestions on TB Prevention and Treatment Work in the Countryside" (对农村肺结核病防治工作的意见). *China Anti-TB Journal* (中国防痨杂志) 7(1): 22–23.

Cui Yitian (崔义田). 1966. *The Work of Sanitation in the First Five-Year Plan* (第一个五年计划中的卫生保健事业) Beijing: All-China Science and Technology Propaganda Association (科学技术普及协会).

Daniel, Thomas M. 2011. "Hermann Brehmer and the Origins of Tuberculosis Sanatoria." *International Journal of Tuberculosis and Lung Disease* 15(2): 161–62.

Davenne, Tamara and Helen McShane. 2016. "Why Don't We Have an Effective Tuberculosis Vaccine Yet?" *Expert Review of Vaccines* 15(8): 1009–13.

Davis, Mike. 2022. *The Monster Enters: Covid-19, Avian Flu, and the Plagues of Capitalism.* London: Verso.

Davis, Noel. 1921. "Health Officer's Report for May." *Municipal Gazette* 14: 231.

Davis, Noel. 1923. "Health Department Report for December (1922)" *Municipal Gazette* 16: 16.

Deng, Wei, Andrew Wilkes, and Gerald Bloom. 1997. "Village Health Services in Rural China." *IDS Bulletin* 28(1): 32–47.

Dikötter, Frank. 2010. *Mao's Great Famine: The History of China's Most Devastating Catastrophe, 1958–1962.* London: Bloomsbury.

Dillon, Nara. 2015. *Radical Inequalities: China's Revolutionary Welfare State in Comparative Perspective.* Cambridge, MA: Harvard East Asian Monographs.

DiMoia, John. 2013. *Reconstructing Bodies: Biomedicine, Nation Building, and Health in South Korea since 1945.* Palo Alto, CA: Stanford University Press.

Dubos, René and Jean Dubos. [1952] 1987. *The White Plague: Tuberculosis, Man, and Society.* New Brunswick, NJ: Rutgers University Press.

Duckett, Jane. 2004. "State, Collectivism and Worker Privilege: A Study of Urban Health Insurance Reform." *China Quarterly* 177: 155–73.

Enarson, Donald A. 2006. "Migrant Tuberculosis: A Moving Target." *International Journal of Tuberculosis and Lung Disease* 10(9): 945.

Eylers, Eva. 2014. "Planning the Nation: The Sanatorium Movement in Germany." *Journal of Architecture* 19(5): 667–92.

Fan Shunhua (范舜华), ed. 1998. *Zhabei Health Gazetteer* (闸北卫生志). Shanghai: Shanghai Youth Daily Publishers (上海市青年报社印刷厂).

Fang, Xiaoping. 2012. *Barefoot Doctors and Western Medicine in China.* Rochester, NY: University of Rochester Press.

Fang, Xiaoping. 2021. *China and the Cholera Pandemic: Restructuring Society under Mao.* Pittsburgh, PA: University of Pittsburgh Press.

Farmer, Paul. 1997. "Social Scientists and the New Tuberculosis." *Social Science & Medicine* 44(3): 347–58.

Farmer, Paul. 2001. *Infections and Inequalities: The Modern Plagues.* Berkeley: University of California Press.

Feldberg, Georgina D. 1995. *Disease and Class: Tuberculosis and the Shaping of Modern American Society.* New Brunswick, NJ: Rutgers University Press.

Feng, Wang, Xuejin Zuo, and Danching Ruan. 2002. "Rural Migrants in Shanghai: Living under the Shadow of Socialism." *International Migration Review* 36(2): 520–45.

References

Fengxian County Health Bureau *Health Gazetteer* Writing Group (奉贤县卫生局《卫生志》编写组). 1985. *Fengxian County Health Gazetteer* (奉贤县卫生志). Shanghai: Fengxian Printing Factory (上海贤奉贤印刷厂).

Festenstein, Freda and John M. Grange. 1999. "Tuberculosis in Ethnic Minority Populations in Industrialized Countries." Pp. 313–38 in *Tuberculosis: An Interdisciplinary Perspective*, edited by J. D. H. Porter and J. M. Grange. London: Imperial College Press.

Foucault, Michel. 2004. *The Birth of Biopolitics: Lectures at the Collège de France*. New York: Picador.

Frazier, Mark W. 2010. *Socialist Insecurity: Pensions and the Politics of Uneven Development in China*. Ithaca, NY: Cornell University Press.

Frieden, Thomas R., Paula I. Fujiwara, Rita M. Washko, and Margaret A. Hamburg. 1995. "Tuberculosis in New York City—Turning the Tide." *New England Journal of Medicine* 333: 229–33.

Fujiwara, Paula I. 2000. "Tide Pools: What Will Be Left after the Tide Has Turned?" *International Journal of Tuberculosis and Lung Disease* 4(12): S111–16.

Furth, Charlotte. 2011. "Introduction: Hygienic Modernity in Chinese East Asia." Pp. 1–24 in *Health and Hygiene in Chinese East Asia*, edited by A. K. C. Leung and C. Furth. Durham, NC: Duke University Press.

Gallagher, Mary. 2005. *Contagious Capitalism: Globalization and the Politics of Labor in China*. Princeton, NJ: Princeton University Press.

Gallagher, Mary, Ching Kwan Lee, and Sarosh Kuruvilla. 2011. "Introduction and Argument." Pp. 1–14 in *From Iron Rice Bowl to Informalization: Markets, Workers, and the State in Changing China*, edited by S. Kuruvilla, C. K. Lee, and M. E. Gallagher. Ithaca, NY: Cornell University Press.

Gamsa, Mark. 2006. "The Epidemic of Pneumonic Plague in Manchuria, 1910–1911." *Past & Present* 190: 147–83.

Gao, Xi. 2014. "Foreign Models of Medicine in Twentieth-Century China." Pp. 173–211 in *Medical Transitions in Twentieth-Century China*, edited by Bridie Andrews and Mary Brown Bullock. Bloomington: University of Indiana Press.

Gardner, John. 1969. "The Wu-Fan Campaign in Shanghai." Pp. 477–539 in *Chinese Communist Politics in Action*, edited by D. Barnett. Seattle: University of Washington Press.

Gewirtz, Julian. 2020. "'Loving Capitalism Disease': AIDS and Ideology in the People's Republic of China, 1984–2000." *Past & Present* 249(1): 251–94. Accessed November 21, 2020 (https://doi.org/10.1093/pastj/gtz068).

Ghandi, Neel, Paul Nunn, Keertan Dheda, Simon Schaaf, Matteo Zignol, Dick van Soolingen, Paul Jensen, and Jamie Bayona. 2010. "Multidrug-Resistant and Extensively Drug-Resistant Tuberculosis: A Threat to Global Control of TB." *Lancet* 375 (May 22): 1830–43.

Ghosh, Arunabh. 2020. *Making It Count: Statistics and Statecraft in the Early People's Republic of China*. Princeton, NJ: Princeton University Press.

Goffman, Erving. 1961. *Asylums: Essays on the Social Situation of Mental Patients and Other Inmates*. New York: Anchor Books.

Golub, Jonathan E., Carolyn I. Mohan, George W. Comstock, and Richard E. Chaisson. 2005. "Active Case Finding of Tuberculosis: Historical Perspective and Future Prospects." *International Journal of Tuberculosis and Lung Disease* 9(11): 1183–203.

Gong You-Long and Chao Li-min. 1982. "The Role of Barefoot Doctors." *American Journal of Public Health* 72 (supplement): 59–62.

Goodman, David S. G. 2014. *Class in Contemporary China*. Cambridge: Polity Press.

Gross, Miriam. 2016. *Farewell to the God of Plague: Chairman Mao's Campaign to Deworm China*. Berkeley: University of California Press.

Gross, Miriam and Kawai Fan. 2014. "Schistosomiasis." Pp. 106–23 in *Medical Transitions in Twentieth Century China*, edited by B. Andrews and M. B. Bullock. Bloomington: University of Indiana Press.

Grypma, Sonya and Cheng Zhen. 2014. "The Development of Modern Nursing in China." Pp. 297–316 in *Medical Transitions in Twentieth-Century China*, edited by B. Andrews and M. B. Bullock. Bloomington: University of Indiana Press.

Gui, Shixun and Liu Xian. 1992. "Urban Migration in Shanghai, 1950–1988: Trends and Characteristics." *Population and Development Review* 18(3): 533–48.

Guttiérrez, John A. 2017. "'An Earnest Pledge to Fight Tuberculosis': Tuberculosis, Nation, and Modernity in Cuba, 1899–1908." *Cuban Studies* 45: 280–96.

Han, Jia-jing and Sheng-ji Yang. 1982. "Tuberculosis Control." *American Journal of Public Health* 72 (Supplement): 48–49.

Hanson, Marta. 2017. "Visualizing the Geography of the Diseases of China: Western Disease Maps from Analytical Tools to Tools of Empire, Sovereignty, and Public Health Propaganda, 1878–1929." *Science in Context* 30(3): 219–80.

Harrison, Mark. 2012. *Contagion: How Commerce Has Spread Disease*. New Haven, CT: Yale University Press.

"Health Department." 1919. *Shanghai Municipal Gazette*, April 11, 122–23.

Henderson, Gail, John Akin, Li Zhiming, Jin Shuigao, Ma Haijiang, and Ge Keyou. 1994. "Equity and the Utilization of Health Services: Report of an Eight-Province Survey in China." *Social Science and Medicine* 39(5): 687–99.

Henderson, Gail E. and Myron S. Cohen. 1984. *The Chinese Hospital: A Socialist Work Unit*. New Haven, CT: Yale University Press.

Henderson, Gail, Suzanne Maman, Yingying Huang, and Suiming Pan. 2014. "Social Contexts of Heterosexual Transmission of HIV/STI in Liuzhou City, China." *AIDS and Behavior* 18 (Supplement 2): 111–17.

Henriot, Christian. 2006. "Shanghai and the Experience of War: The Fate of Refugees." *European Journal of East Asian Studies* 5(2): 215–45.

Henriot, Christian. 2009. "'Invisible Deaths, Silent Deaths': 'Bodies without Masters' in Republican Shanghai." *Journal of Social History* 43(2): 407–37.

Henriot, Christian. 2016. *Scythe and the City: A Social History of Death in Shanghai*. Stanford, CA: Stanford University Press.

Hillier, Sheila and J. Anthony Jewell. 1983. *Health and Traditional Medicine in China, 1800–1982*. London: Routledge and Kegan Paul.

Ho, Denise Y. 2017. *Curating Revolution: Politics on Display in Mao's China*. Cambridge: Cambridge University Press.

References

Ho, Ming-Jung. 2004. "Sociocultural Aspects of Tuberculosis: A Literature Review and a Case Study of Immigrant Tuberculosis." *Social Science & Medicine* 59(4): 753–62.

Honig, Emily. 1986. *Sisters and Strangers: Women in the Shanghai Cotton Mills, 1919–1949.* Stanford, CA: Stanford University Press.

Horn, Joshua. 1971. *Away with All Pests: An English Surgeon in People's China, 1954–69.* New York: Monthly Review Press.

Howe, Christopher. 1971. *Employment and Economic Growth in Urban China, 1949–57.* New York: Cambridge University Press.

Howe, Christopher. 1981. "Industrialization under Conditions of Long-Run Population Stability: Shanghai's Achievement and Prospect." Pp. 153–87 in *Shanghai: Revolution and Development in an Asian Metropolis,* edited by C. Howe. New York: Cambridge University Press.

Howlett, Jonathan J. 2013. "'The British Boss Is Gone and Will Never Return': Communist Takeovers of British Companies in Shanghai (1949–1954)." *Modern Asian Studies* 47(6): 1941–76.

Hsu, Robert C. 1974. "The Barefoot Doctors of the People's Republic of China—Some Problems." *New England Journal of Medicine.* 291(3): 124–27.

Hu, Richard and Weijie Chen. 2019. *Global Shanghai Remade: The Rise of Pudong New Area.* Milton, MA: Taylor & Francis.

Huang, Philip. 1990. *The Peasant Family and Rural Development in the Yangzi Delta, 1350–1988.* Stanford, CA: Stanford University Press.

"Humorous Reading" (幽默读). 1958. *Combat Tuberculosis* (抗痨) 162 (February 1): 7.

Hung, Chang-tai. 2011. *Mao's New World: Political Culture in the Early People's Republic.* Ithaca, NY: Cornell University Press.

Hung, Chang-tai. 2021. *Politics of Control: Creating Red Culture in the Early People's Republic of China.* Honolulu: University of Hawai'i Press.

Hyde, Sandra Teresa. 2007. *Eating Spring Rice: The Cultural Politics of AIDS in Southwest China.* Berkeley: University of California Press.

Jackson, Isabella. 2012. "Managing Shanghai: The International Settlement Administration and the Development of the City." PhD dissertation, University of Bristol.

Jackson, Isabella. 2017. *Shaping Modern Shanghai: Colonialism in China's Global City.* Cambridge: Cambridge University Press.

Jain-Chandra, Sonali, Tidiane Kinda, Kalpana Kochhar, Shi Piao, and Johanna Schauer. 2016. "Sharing the Growth Dividend: Analysis of Inequality in Asia." International Monetary Fund Working Paper (WP/16/48). Accessed June 6, 2018 (https://www.imf.org/en/Publications/WP/Issues/2016/12/31/Sharing-the-Growth-Dividend-Analysis-of-Inequality-in-Asia-43767).

Jaramillo, Ernesto. 1999. "Encompassing Treatment with Prevention: The Path for a Lasting Control of Tuberculosis." *Social Science & Medicine* 49: 393–404.

Jaros, Kyle A. 2019. *China's Urban Champions: The Politics of Spatial Development.* Princeton, NJ: Princeton University Press.

Jewell, Tony. 1996. "Authors Overestimate Role of Barefoot Doctors in China." *British Medical Journal* 312: 250.

Jiading Health Gazetteer Compilation Committee (嘉定卫生志编纂委员会). 2011. *Jiading Health Gazetteer* (嘉定卫生). Shanghai: Xuelin Publishing House. (学林出版社).

Jinshan County Health Gazetteer editorial members (金山县卫生志编纂成员), eds. 1994. *Jinshan County Health Gazetteer* (金山县卫生志). Shanghai: Shanghai Children's Publishing Service (上海少儿出版服务社).

Johnson, Matthew. 2015. "Beneath the Propaganda State: Official and Unofficial Cultural Landscapes in Shanghai, 1949–1965." Pp. 199–229 in *Maoism at the Grassroots: Everyday Life in China's Era of High Socialism*, edited by J. Brown and M. Johnson. Cambridge, MA: Harvard University Press.

Johnston, William. 1995. *The Modern Epidemic: A History of Tuberculosis in Japan*. Cambridge, MA: Harvard University Press.

Jordan, J. H. 1928. "Health Officer's Report for April." *Municipal Gazette* 20: 210.

Kerrigan, Amanda L. 2018. "Medical Protests in China: How China's One-Party System Adapts to Social Conflict." PhD dissertation, Johns Hopkins University.

Keshavjee, Salmaan. 2014. *Blind Spot: How Neoliberalism Infiltrated Global Health*. Berkeley: University of California Press.

Knopf, S. Adolphus. 1922. *A History of the National Tuberculosis Association: The Antituberculosis Movement in the United States*. New York: National Tuberculosis Association.

Koch, Erin. 2013. *Free Market Tuberculosis: Managing Epidemics in Post-Soviet Georgia*. Nashville, TN: Vanderbilt University Press.

Koplan, Jeffrey, Alan Hinman, Robert Parker, You-Long Gong, and Ming-Ding Yang. 1985. "The Barefoot Doctor: Shanghai County Revisited." *American Journal of Public Health* 75(7): 768–70.

Lam, Tong. 2011. *A Passion for Facts: Social Surveys and the Construction of the Chinese Nation-State, 1900–1949*. Berkeley: University of California Press.

LaMotte, Ellen N. 1908. "Some Phases of the Tuberculosis Question." *American Journal of Nursing* 8(6): 430–34.

Lei, Sean Hsiang-lin. 2010. "Habituating Individuality: The Framing of Tuberculosis and Its Material Solutions in Republican China." *Bulletin of the History of Medicine* 84: 248–79.

Lei, Sean Hsiang-lin. 2014. *Neither Donkey nor Horse: Medicine in the Struggle over China's Modernity*. Chicago: University of Chicago.

Leung, Joe. 1994. "Dismantling the 'Iron Rice Bowl': Welfare Reforms in the People's Republic of China." *Journal of Social Policy* 23(3): 341–61.

Li Hengjun (李恒俊). 2014. "Tuberculosis in Modern China: A Social and Cultural History (1850–1940s)" (疾病知识、医疗文化与卫生现代性: 近代中国肺结核病的社会与文化史). PhD dissertation, National University of Singapore.

Li, Jie. 2020. "Revolutionary Echoes: Radios and Loudspeakers in the Mao Era." *Twentieth Century China* 45(1): 25–45.

Li, Ting'an. 1934. "Summary Report on Rural Public Health Practice in China." *Chinese Medical Journal* 48 (October): 1086–90.

Li, Ting'an. 1935. "Activities of the Bureau of Public Health, City Government of Greater Shanghai." *Chinese Medical Journal* 49: 990–92.

Li, Victor H. 1975. "Politics and Health Care in China: The Barefoot Doctors." *Stanford Law Review* 27(827): 827–40.

References

Lin, Kevin. 2015. "Recomposing Chinese Migrant and State-Sector Workers." Pp. 68–84 in *Chinese Workers in Comparative Perspective*, edited by A. Chan. Ithaca, NY: Cornell University Press.

Link, Bruce and Jo Phelan. 1995. "Social Conditions as Fundamental Causes of Disease." *Journal of Health and Social Behavior* 35 (extra issue): 80–94.

Liu, Gordon G. and Sam Krumholz. 2017. "Epidemiological Transition and Health System Reforms in China." *China's Healthcare System and Reforms*. Pp. 119–36 in *China's Healthcare System and Reform*, edited by L. R. Burns and G. G. Liu. New York: Cambridge University Press.

Liu Qiong (刘琼), ed. 2011. *Xinqiao Town Gazetteer* (新桥镇志) Shanghai Dictionary Publishers (上海辞书出版社).

Liu Qiong and Hui Yu (刘琼, 蕙郁), eds. 2012. *Sheshan Town Gazetteer* (佘山镇志). Shanghai Dictionary Publishers (上海辞书出版社).

Liu, Yuanli, William C. L. Hsiao, Qing Li, Xingzhu Liu, and Minghui Ren. 1995. "Transformation of China's Rural Health Care Financing." *Social Science & Medicine* 41(8): 1085–93.

Liu, Shao-hua. 2011. *Passage to Manhood: Youth Migration, Heroin, and AIDS in Southwest China*. Stanford, CA: Stanford University Press.

Long, Qian, Yan Qu, and Henry Lucas. 2016. "Drug-Resistant Tuberculosis Control in China: Progress and Challenges." Figshare. Accessed October 10, 2020 (https://search.datacite.org/works/10.6084/m9.figshare.c.3639347).

Lu, Hanchao. 1999. *Beyond the Neon Lights: Everyday Shanghai in the Early Twentieth Century*. Berkeley: University of California Press.

Lu, Liping, Qi Jiang, Jianjun Hong, Xiaoping Jin, Qian Gao, Heejung Bang, Kathryn DeRiemer, and Chongguang Yang. 2020. "Catastrophic Costs of Tuberculosis Care in a Population with Internal Migrants in China." *BMC Health Services Research* 20: 832.

Lu, Ming, and Yiran Xia. 2016. "Migration in the People's Republic of China." *ADBI Working Paper 593*. Tokyo: Asian Development Bank Institute. Accessed May 20, 2021 (https://www.adb.org/publications/migration-people-republic-china/).

Lü, Xiaobo and Elizabeth J. Perry. 1997. "Introduction: The Changing Chinese Workplace in Historical and Comparative Perspective." Pp. 3–17 in *Danwei*, edited by X. Lü and E. J. Perry. Armonk, NY: M. E. Sharpe.

Lü Xuetong (陆学通). 1990. *Shanghai County Health Gazetteer* (上海县卫生志). Shanghai: Shanghai County Health Bureau (上海县卫生局).

Lu Xun. [1922] 1972. "Medicine." *Selected Stories of Lu Hsun*. Beijing: Foreign Languages Press.

Lucas, Anelissa. 1980. "Changing Medical Models in China: Organizational Options or Obstacles?" *China Quarterly* 83: 461–89.

Lynteris, Christos. 2013. "Skilled Natives, Inept Coolies: Marmot Hunting and the Great Manchurian Pneumonic Plague (1910–1911)." *History and Anthropology* 24(3): 303–12.

Lynteris, Christos. 2018. "Plague Masks: The Visual Emergence of Anti-Epidemic Personal Protection Equipment" *Medical Anthropology* 37(6): 442–57.

MacPherson, Kerrie L. 1987. *A Wilderness of Marshes: The Origins of Public Health in Shanghai, 1843 1893*. Hong Kong: Oxford University Press.

MacPherson, Kerrie L. 1990. "Designing China's Urban Future: The Greater Shanghai Plan, 1927–37." *Planning Perspective* 5(1): 39–62.

Marmott, Michael. 2004. *The Status Syndrome: How Social Standing Affects Our Health and Longevity*. New York: Henry Holt.

Mason, Katherine. 2016. *Infectious Change: Reinventing Chinese Public Health after an Epidemic*. Stanford, CA: Stanford University Press.

McKee, Martin. 2005. "Monitoring Health in Central and Eastern Europe and the Former Soviet Union." *Social and Preventative Medicine* 50(6): 341–43.

McKeown, Thomas. 1976. *The Modern Rise of Population*. New York: Academic Press.

McMillen, Christian W. 2015. *Discovering Tuberculosis: A Global History, 1900 to the Present*. New Haven, CT: Yale University Press.

McMillen, Christian W. and Niels Brimnes. 2010. "Medical Modernization and Medical Nationalism: Resistance to Mass Tuberculosis Vaccination in Postcolonial India, 1948–1955." *Comparative Studies in Society and History* 52(1): 180–209.

McNeill, William H. 1977. *Plagues and People*. New York: Anchor Books.

Mei Yulin, Zhong Zhesheng, and Wang Wenzhen (梅玉麟, 衷浙生, 王文珍), eds. 1991. *Chronicle of the Xuhui District TB and Lung Tumor Prevention and Treatment Clinic* (徐汇区结核病肺部肿防治所所志). Shanghai: n.p.

Mera, Frank E. 1935. "History of the Sanatorium Movement in America." *Diseases of the Chest* 1(1): 8–9.

Michaels, Paula A. 2003. *Curative Powers: Medicine and Empire in Stalin's Central Asia*. Pittsburgh, PA: University of Pittsburgh Press.

Molero-Mesa, Jorge. 2010. "'The Right Not to Suffer Consumption': Health, Welfare Charity, and the Working Class in Spain." Pp. 171–82 in *TB Then and Now: Perspectives on the History of Infectious Disease*, edited by Flurin Condrau and Michael Worboys. Montreal: McGill-Queen's University Press.

"Municipal Gaol—Dietary." 1922. *Municipal Gazette*, December 21, 448–50.

Murphey, Rhoads. 1953. *Shanghai: Key to Modern China*. Cambridge, MA: Harvard University Press.

Nakajima, Cheiko. 2018. *Body, Society, and Nation: The Creation of Public Health and Urban Culture in Shanghai*. Cambridge, MA: Harvard University Asia Center.

Nanhui Health Gazetteer Writing Leadership Team (南汇县卫生志编写领导小组). 1987. *Nanhui Health Gazetteer* (南汇县卫生志). Shanghai: n.p.

National Anti-Tuberculosis Association of China (中国防痨协会). n.d. "Hidden Disaster" (祸隐). Shanghai: n.p.

Navarro, Vicente. 2007. *Globalization and Inequalities: Consequences for Health and Quality of Life*. Amityville, NY: Baywood.

New, Peter Kong-Ming and Mary Louie New. 1975. "The Links between Health and Political Structure in New China." *Human Organization* 34(3): 237–51.

Oi, Jean C. 1999. *Rural China Takes Off: Institutional Foundations of Economic Reform*. Berkeley: University of California Press.

References

199

Okeke, Iruka, Adebayo Lamikanra, and Robert Edelman. 1999. "Socioeconomic and Behavioral Factors Leading to Acquired Bacterial Resistance to Antibiotics in Developing Countries." *Emerging Infectious Diseases* 5(1): 1999.

Ott, Katherine. 1996. *Fevered Lives: Tuberculosis in American Culture since 1970*. Cambridge, MA: Harvard University Press.

Packard, Randall. 1989. *White Plague, Black Labor: Tuberculosis and the Political Economy of Health and Disease in South Africa*. Berkeley: University of California Press.

Packard, Randall. 2016. *A History of Global Health: Interventions into the Lives of Other Peoples*. Baltimore: Johns Hopkins University Press.

Park, Albert and Fang Cai. 2011. "The Informalization of the Chinese Labor Market." Pp. 17–35 in *From Iron Rice Bowl to Informalization: Markets, Workers, and the State in Changing China*, edited by S. Kuruvilla, C. K. Lee, and M. E. Gallagher. Ithaca, NY: Cornell University Press.

Patriotic Hygiene Committee (爱国卫生运动). 1953. *Hygiene Propaganda Education* (卫生宣传教育), edited by Dong Junjing (董俊菁). Beijing: People's Hygiene Press (人民卫生出版社).

Peng, Jing, Shengnian Zhang, Wei Lu, and Andrew T. L. Chen. 2003. "Public Health in China: The Shanghai CDC Perspective." *American Journal of Public Health* 93(12): 1991–93.

Perkins, James A. 1954. "The National Tuberculosis Association." *Public Health Reports* 69(5): 513–18.

Permanyer, Iñaki and Jeroen Smits. 2018. "The Subnational Human Development Index: Moving beyond Country-Level Averages." *United Nations Development Program Human Development Reports*. Accessed June 6, 2018 (https://globaldatalab.org/shdi/).

Perry, Elizabeth. 2002. "Moving the Masses: Emotion Work in the Chinese Revolution." *Mobilization* 7(2): 111–28.

Pickowicz, Paul G. 1971. "Barefoot Doctors in China: People, Politics, and Paramedicine." *Eastern Horizon* 11: 25–38.

Porter, Dorothy. 1999. *Health, Civilization and the State: A History of Public Health from Ancient to Modern Times*. New York: Routledge.

Qian, Dongfu, Henry Lucas, Jiaying Chen, Ling Xu, and Yaoguang Zhang. 2010. "Determinants of the Use of Different Types of Health Care Provider in Urban China." *Health Policy* 98: 227–35.

Qian, Zengwei and Zhang Yuming (钱曾玮, 张玉铭). 1985. "Initial Report on Songjiang County TB Monitoring Work" (松江县结核病监测工作初抱). *China Anti-TB Journal* (中国防痨通讯) 7(4): 155–56.

Qiao, Zhengyue. 2020. "A Hospital That Spearheaded the City's Tuberculosis Fight in 1920s." *Shine beyond a Single Story*. Accessed December 30, 2020 (https://www.shine.cn/feature/art-culture/2009045444/).

Qingpu Health Gazetteer Compilation Committee (青浦县卫生志编纂委员会). 1989. *Qingpu Health Gazetteer* (青浦县卫生志). Shanghai: Shanghai Science and Technology Press (上海科学技术出版社).

Raviglione, Mark and Antonio Poi. 2002 "Evolution of WHO Policies for Tuberculosis Control, 1948–2001." *Lancet* 359: 775–80.

"Resolution VII." 1914. *Municipal Gazette*, March 21, 96–98.

Rifkin, Susan B. 1978. " Politics of Barefoot Medicine." *Lancet* 311 (8054): 34.

Riis, Jacob. 1890. *How the Other Half Lives*. New York: Scribner.

Riis, Jacob. 1893. "Police Lodging Houses: Are They Hotbeds for Typhus?" *Christian Union*, January 14. Part of the Library of Congress Online Exhibit, *Jacob Riis: Revealing How the Other Half Lives*. Accessed June 15, 2021 (https://www.loc.gov/exhibits/jacob-riis/reporter.html#obj050).

Riis, Jacob. 1907. "The Christmas Stamp." *Outlook* 86(10): 511–14.

Ristaino, Marcia. 2008. *The Jaquinot Safe Zone: Wartime Refugees in Shanghai*. Palo Alto, CA: Stanford University Press.

Roberts, Samuel Kelton, Jr. 2009. *Infectious Fear: Politics, Disease, and the Health Effects of Segregation*. Chapel Hill: University of North Carolina Press.

Rogaski, Ruth. 2002. "Nature, Annihilation, and Modernity: China's Korean War Germ-Warfare Experience Reconsidered." *Journal of Asian Studies* 61(2): 381–415.

Rogaski, Ruth. 2004. *Hygienic Modernity: Meanings of Health and Disease in Treaty Port China*. Berkeley: University of California Press.

Rogaski, Ruth. 2022. *Knowing Manchuria: Environments, Senses, and Natural Knowledge on an Asian Borderland*. Chicago: University of Chicago Press.

Rosen, George. 1993. *A History of Public Health*. 2nd ed. Baltimore: Johns Hopkins University Press.

Rothman, Sheila. 1994. *Living in the Shadow of Death: Tuberculosis and the Social Experience of Illness in American History*. Baltimore: Johns Hopkins University Press.

Sanitize, Eka and Ramaz Shengelia. 2015. "First Partnerships to Fight Tuberculosis." *Journal of Clinical Research & Bioethics* 6(5): 241. Accessed February 28, 2022 (https://doi.org/10.4172/2155-9627.1000241).

Sassen, Saskia. 1991. *The Global City: New York, London, Tokyo*. Princeton, NJ: Princeton University Press.

Sassen, Saskia. 2005. "The Global City: Introducing a Concept." *Brown Journal of World Affairs* 11(2): 27–43.

Scheid, Volker. 2002. *Chinese Medicine in Contemporary China: Plurality and Synthesis*. Durham, NC: Duke University Press.

Schmalzer, Sigrid. 2016. *Red Revolution, Green Revolution: Scientific Farming in Socialist China*. Chicago: University of Chicago Press.

Shandong Provincial Health Gazetteer Editorial Committee (山东省卫生史志编纂委员会). 1991. *Shandong Provincial Health Gazetteer* (山东省卫生志). Jinan: Shandong People's Press.

Shanghai Anti-Tuberculosis Association (SATA). 1942. "Campaign for the Support of Free Tuberculosis Hospitalization & Free Tuberculosis Clinic Treatment." *SATA Bulletin* 1(10–12): 17–23.

Shanghai Anti-Tuberculosis Association (上海防痨协会, SATA). 1953a. *Shanghai Anti-Tuberculosis Association 1952 Annual Report* (上海防痨协会一九五二年年报). Shanghai: n.p.

Shanghai Anti-Tuberculosis Association (上海防痨协会, SATA). 1953b. "SATA's 1952 Work Summary" (上海防痨协会1952年工作总结). *Anti-TB Journal* (防痨通讯) 6(2): 1–5.

Shanghai Anti-Tuberculosis Association (上海防痨协会, SATA). 1953–1954. United States National Library of Medicine Chinese Public Health Collection (US NLM CPHC). Accessed August 22, 2022 (https://www.nlm.nih.gov/exhibition/chinesean-titb/fourseries4.html).

Shanghai Health Bureau Prevention Office (上海市卫生局医疗预防处). 1958. "Shanghai Municipal TB Prevention and Treatment Work during the GLF" (上海市结核病防治工作在跃进中). *China Anti-Tuberculosis* (中国防痨) 1(4): 10.

Shanghai Municipal Archives (SMA, 上海市档案馆) files: B123-8-1055-22, B168-1-818, B242-1-194, B242-1-530, B242-1-535-60, B242-1-1176, B242-1-1510, B242-3-754-132, Q199-20-43, Q400-1-4053, R50-1-140, U1-16-148, U1-16-617, U1-16-654, U1-16-655, U1-16-656, U1-16-617, U1-16-714, U1-16-2659, U1-16-2660, U1-16-2661, U1-16-2662, U1-16-2663, U1-16-2664, U1-16-2665, U38-1-191, U38-1-192, U38-5-1091, U38-5-1625.

Shanghai Municipal Council (SMC). 1913. *Report for the Year 1912 and Budget for the Year 1913*. Shanghai: Kelly and Walsh.

Shanghai Municipal Council (SMC). 1920. *Report for the Year 1919 and Budget for the Year 1920*. Shanghai: Kelly and Walsh.

Shanghai Municipal Council (SMC). 1922. *Report for the Year 1921 and Budget for the Year 1922*. Shanghai: Kelly and Walsh.

Shanghai Science and Technology Press (上海科学技术出版社), ed. 1959. *Shanghai Hygiene: Experience of First Entering the Work Units* (上海卫生先进单位的经验). Shanghai: Science and Technology Press (上海科学技术出版社).

Shanghai Statistical Yearbook Editorial Committee (上海统计年鉴编辑委员会). 2004. *2004 Shanghai Statistical Yearbook* (2004上海统计年鉴). Beijing: China Statistics Press (中国统计出版社).

Shanghai Statistical Yearbook Editorial Committee (上海统计年鉴编辑委员会). 2008. *2008 Shanghai Statistical Yearbook* (2008上海统计年鉴). Beijing: China Statistics Press (中国统计出版社).

Shanghai Statistical Yearbook Editorial Committee (上海统计年鉴编辑委员会). 2010. *2010 Shanghai Statistical Yearbook* (2010上海统计年鉴). Beijing: China Statistics Press (中国统计出版社).

Shanghai Statistical Yearbook Editorial Committee (上海统计年鉴编辑委员会). 2017. *2017 Shanghai Statistical Yearbook* (2017上海统计年鉴). Beijing: China Statistics Press (中国统计出版社).

Shanghai Yangpu District Gazetteer Compilation Committee (上海市杨浦区地方志编纂委员会). 2009. *1991–2003 Yangpu District Gazetteer* (杨浦区志1991–2003). Shanghai: Shanghai Higher Education Electronic Audio and Video Press (上海高教电子音像出版社).

Shapiro, Judith. 2001. *Mao's War against Nature: Politics and the Environment in Revolutionary China*. New York: Cambridge University Press.

Shen, Xin, Zhen Xia, Xiangqun Li, Jie Wu, Lili Wang, Jing Li, Yuan Jiang, Juntao Guo, Jing Chen, Jianjun Hong, Zhang'an Yuan, Qichao Pan, Kathryn DeRiemer, Guomei Sun, Qian Gao, and Jian Mei. 2012. "Tuberculosis in an Urban Area in China: Differences between Urban Migrants and Local Residents." *PLoS One* 7(1): e51133.

Shirk, Susan. 1993. *The Political Logic of Economic Reform in China*. Berkeley: University of California Press.

Sidel, Ruth and Victor W. Sidel. 1977. "Health Services." *Social Scientist* 5(10/11): 114–30.

Sidel, Victor W. and Ruth Sidel. 1974. *Serve the People: Observations in the People's Republic of China*. Boston: Beacon Press.

Sidel, Victor W. and Ruth Sidel. 1982. *The Health of China*. Boston: Beacon Press.

Sinclair, Upton. 1906. *The Jungle*. New York: Doubleday.

Solinger, Dorothy. 1997. "The Impact of the Floating Population on the *Danwei*: Shifts in the Patterns of Labor Mobility Control and Entitlement Provision." Pp. 192–222 in *Danwei: The Changing Chinese Workplace in Historical and Comparative Perspective*, edited by X. Lü and E. J. Perry. Armonk, NY: M. E. Sharpe.

Solinger, Dorothy. 1999. *Contesting Citizenship in Urban China: Peasant Migrants, the State, and the Logic of Market*. Berkeley: University of California Press.

Song Yandong (宋延栋). 1953. "First Anti-TB Focal Point Testing: Initial Results of TB Promotion Work at the Fifth National Cotton Factory." (下厂防痨的一个重点试验：上海国棉五厂推行防痨工作初步总结) *Shanghai Anti-TB* (上海防痨) 3(6): 6–10.

Song Yandong and Chen Weitang (宋延栋, 陈维糖). 1954. "One Factory's Harvest from a Year of Anti-TB Work" (一年来工厂防痨工作的收获). *Shanghai Anti-TB* (上海防痨) 4(6): 1–3.

Song Yandong and Chen Weitang (宋延栋, 陈维糖). 1956. "Initial Opinion on Two Previous Years of Anti TB Results in Shanghai's Fifth National Cotton Factory" (上海国棉五厂两年来防痨效果的初步观察). *Anti-TB Journal* (防痨通讯) 9(5): 1–3.

Soon, Wayne. 2020. *Global Medicine in China: A Diasporic History*. Redwood City, CA: Stanford University Press.

Soon, Wayne and Ja Ian Chong. 2020. "What History Teaches about the Coronavirus Emergency: Lessons of Transparency and Transnational Cooperation from the 1910–1911 Manchurian Plague Are Still Relevant to China and the World Today." *Diplomat*, February 12. Accessed June 22, 2021 (https://thediplomat.com/2020/02/what-history-teaches-about-the-wuhan-coronavirus/).

Stanley, Arthur. 1909. "Health Officer's Report for March." *Municipal Gazette* 2: 124.

Stanley, Arthur. 1912. "Health Officer's Report for March." *Municipal Gazette* 5: 123.

Stanley, Arthur. 1913a. "Health Officer's Report for September." *Municipal Gazette* 6: 241.

Stanley, Arthur. 1913b. "Health Officer's Report for October." *Municipal Gazette* 6: 260.

Stanley, Arthur. 1913c. "Health Officer's Report for November." *Municipal Gazette* 6: 292.

Stanley, Arthur. 1917. "Health Officer's Report for April." *Municipal Gazette* 10: 153.

Stanley, Arthur. 1918a. "Health Officer's Report for January." *Municipal Gazette* 11: 50.

Stanley, Arthur. 1918b. "Health Officer's Report for April." *Municipal Gazette* 11: 166–67.

Stanley, Arthur. 1919a. "Health Officer's Report for March." *Municipal Gazette* 12: 146–47.

Stanley, Arthur. 1919b. "Health Officer's Report for August." *Municipal Gazette* 12: 313.

Stanley, Arthur. 1920c. "Health Officer's Report for April." *Municipal Gazette* 13: 206.

Stanley, Arthur. 1920a. "Health Officer's Report for August." *Municipal Gazette* 13: 324.

Stanley, Arthur. 1920b. "Health Officer's Report for October." *Municipal Gazette* 13: 379.

Stanley, Arthur. 1921. "Health Officer's Report for January." *Municipal Gazette* 14: 47–48.

References

Strachan, Louis. 1933. "The National Tuberculosis Association." *Journal of Health and Physical Education* 4(6): 8–45.

Strauss, Julia. 2006. "Introduction: In Search of PRC History." *China Quarterly* 188: 855–69.

Stuckler, David, Lawrence King, and Martin McKee. 2009. "Mass Privatization and the Post-Communist Mortality Crisis: A Cross-National Analysis." *Lancet* 373: 399–407.

"Suggested Consumption Hospital." 1913. *Municipal Gazette*, October 2, 227–29.

Sun Zhongliang (孙忠亮). 1981. "Shanghai's Prevention and Treatment Situation with Suggestions" (上海结核病防治近况与几点意见). *Bulletin of the China Anti-Tuberculosis Association* (中国防痨通讯) 3(1): 4–7.

Swider, Sarah. 2015. *Building China: Informal Work and the New Precariat*. Ithaca, NY: Cornell University Press.

Sze, Szeming. 1937–1938. "Medical Care for Shanghai Refugees." *China Quarterly* 3 (Winter): 77–83.

Szreter, Simon. 1988. "The Importance of Social Intervention in Britain's Mortality Decline c. 1850–1914: A Re-interpretation of the Role of Public Health." *Social History of Medicine* 1(1): 1–38.

Summers, William C. 2012. *The Great Manchurian Plague of 1910–11: The Geopolitics of an Epidemic Disease*. New Haven, CT: Yale University Press.

Tang, Shenlang, Hana Brixi, and Henk Bekedam. 2014. "Advancing Universal Coverage of Healthcare in China: Translating Political Will into Policy and Practice." *International Journal of Health Planning and Management* 29: 160–74.

Tang, Shenglan and Qingyue Meng. 2004. "Introduction to the Urban Health System and Review of Reform Initiatives." Pp. 17–38 in *Health Care Transition in Urban China*, edited by Gerald Bloom and Shenlang Tang. Burlington, VT: Ashgate.

Taylor, Kim. 2005. *Chinese Medicine in Early Communist China, 1945–1963: A Medicine of Revolution*. London: RoutledgeCurzon.

Teller, Michael A. 1988. *The Tuberculosis Movement: A Public Health Movement in the Progressive Era*. Westport, CT: Greenwood.

Tillman, Margaret Mih. 2018. *Raising China's Revolutionaries: Modernizing Childhood for Cosmopolitan Nationals and Liberated Comrades, 1920s–1950s*. New York: Columbia University Press.

Toman, Kurt. 1979. *Tuberculosis Case Finding and Chemotherapy: Questions and Answers*. Geneva: World Health Organization.

Tu, Jiong. 2019. *Health Care Transformation in Contemporary China: Moral Experience in a Socialist Neoliberal Polity*. Singapore: Springer Nature.

"Tuberculosis Hospital." 1915. *Municipal Gazette*, March 16, 93–95.

Tucker, Joseph D., Xiang-Sheng Chen, and Rosanna W. Peeling. 2010. "Syphilis and Social Upheaval in China." *New England Journal of Medicine* 362(18): 1658–61.

U, Eddy. 2007. *Disorganizing China: Counter-bureaucracy and the Decline of Socialism*. Stanford, CA: Stanford University Press.

Wang, Fei-Ling. 2005. *Organizing through Division and Exclusion: China's Hukou System*. Stanford, CA: Stanford University Press.

Wang Jianxiang and Chen Guyong (王建祥, 陈国勇). 2004. "TB Control Enters Basic Rural Health Protection Practice" (结核病控制纳入农村初级卫生保健实). *China Anti-TB Journal* (中国防痨杂志) 16(4): 150–51.

Wang Jihong (网继红), ed. 2004. *Fengxian County Health Gazetteer* (奉贤县卫生志). Shanghai: Shanghai Century Publishing Stock Company, Ltd. (上海世纪出版股份有限公司).

Wang, Li, Zhihao Wang, Qinglian Ma, Guixia Fang, and Jinxia Yang. 2019. "The Development and Reform of Public Health in China from 1949 to 2019." *Globalization and Health* 15: 45.

Wang, Longde, Jianjun Liu, and Daniel P. Chin. 2007. "Progress in Tuberculosis Control and the Evolving Public-Health System in China." *Lancet* 369(February 24): 691–96.

Wang, Shaoguang. 2004. "China's Health System: From Crisis to Opportunity." *Yale China Health Journal* 3: 5–49.

Wang, Weibing, Qingwu Jiang, Abo Saleh M. Abdullah, and Biao Xu. 2007. "Barriers in Access to Tuberculosis Care among Non-residents in Shanghai: A Descriptive Study of Delays in Diagnosis." *European Journal of Public Health* 17(5): 419.

Wang, Yu, Tanghong Jia, Jinghui Zhang, Yunli Zhang, Wen Li, and Robert Haining. 2012. "Community Health Services in Urban China: A Geographical Case Study of Access to Care." Pp. 164–81 in *Health Care Reform and Globalization: The U.S., China, and Europe in Comparative Perspective*, edited by P. Watson. London: Taylor & Francis.

Wang Yun (王郓). 1952. "On the Advantages of Workers' Insurance" (记 "劳动保险" 给一个工厂厨司带来的幸福). *Health News* (健康报), January 31.

Wang, Zuoye. 2015. "The Chinese Developmental State during the Cold War: The Making of the 1956 Twelve-Year Science and Technology Plan." *History & Technology* 31(3): 180–205.

Watts, Jonathan. 2008. "Chen Zhu: From Barefoot Doctor to China's Minister of Health." *Lancet* 372: 1455.

Wei, Deng, Andreas Wilkes, and Gerald Bloom. 1997. "Village Health Services in Rural China." *IDS Bulletin* 28(1): 32–38.

Wei, Xiaolin, Jing Chen, Ping Chen, James N. Newell, Hongdi Li, Chenguang Sun, Jian Mei, and John D. Walley. 2009. "Barriers to TB Care for Rural-to-Urban Migrant TB Patients in Shanghai: A Qualitative Study." *Tropical Medicine and International Health* 14(7): 754–60.

Whiting, Susan. 2001. *Power and Wealth in Rural China: The Political Economy of Rural Change*. Cambridge: Cambridge University Press.

Whyte, Martin King, and William L. Parish. 1984. *Urban Life in Contemporary China*. Chicago: University of Chicago Press.

Wong, Chack-kie, Vai lo Lo, and Kwong-Leung Tang. 2006. *China's Urban Health Care Reform*. Lanham, MD: Lexington Books.

Wong, K. Chimin and Lien-teh Wu. 1936. *History of Chinese Medicine: Being a Chronicle of Medical Happenings in China from Ancient Times to the Present Period*. Shanghai: National Quarantine Service.

World Bank. n.d. "Life Expectancy at Birth, Total (Years)—China." Accessed June 22, 2022 (https://data.worldbank.org/indicator/SP.DYN.LE00.IN?locations=CN).

References

World Health Organization (WHO). 1999. *What Is DOTS?* Geneva: World Health Organization. Accessed April 15, 2020 (https://apps.who.int/iris/handle/10665/65979).

World Health Organization (WHO). 2019. *Global Tuberculosis Control Report 2019*. Washington, DC.

Wu Shaoqing (吴绍青. 1947. "From Maternal Education to TB Prevention." (从接生教育谈到访痨) *Shanghai Hygiene* (上海卫生) 5(1): 31–32.

Wu Shaoqing (吴绍青). 1949. "Forecasting 38 Years of Work" (三十八年工作之展望) *Anti-TB Journal* (防痨通讯) 2(1): 1.

Wu Shaoqing (吴绍青). 1952. "How Does Shanghai Prevent TB?" (上海如何防痨？). *Shanghai Hygiene* (上海卫生) 2(1): 34–36.

Xiao, Wenming and Yao Li. 2020. "Building a 'Lofty, Beloved People's Amusement Centre': The Socialist Transformation of Shanghai's Great World (Dashijie), 1950–58." *Modern Asian Studies* 55(3): 973–1014.

Xinhua (新华社). 1963. "Conference on TB Control and Research Experience Exchange" (结核病学术会议交流防治和研究经验). *People's Daily* (人民日报), June 30.

Xinhua. 2019. "Shanghai Home to over 700 Regional Headquarters of Multinational Corporations." *China Daily*. Accessed May 21, 2020 (https://www.chinadaily.com.cn/a/201909/15/WS5d7e022ca310cf3e3556b7cd.html).

Xue, Hao, Jennifer Hager, Qi An, Kai Liu, Jing Zhang, Emma Auden, Bingyan Yang, Jie Yang, Hongyan Liu, Jingchun Nie, Aiqin Wang, Chengchao Zhou, Yaojiang Shi, and Sean Sylvia, 2018. "The Quality of Tuberculosis Care in Urban Migrant Clinics in China." *International Journal of Environmental Research and Public Health* 15(9): 2037. Accessed October 10, 2020 (https://doi.org/10.3390/ijerph15092037).

Yan, Zhongmin. 1985. "Shanghai: The Growth and Shifting Emphasis of China's Largest City." Pp. 94–127 in *Chinese Cities: The Growth of the Metropolis since 1949*, edited by Victor F. S. Sit. Oxford: Oxford University Press.

Yang, Dali. 1996. *Calamity and Reform in China: State, Rural Society, and Institutional Change since the Great Leap Famine*. Stanford, CA: Stanford University Press.

Yang, Yansui and Dan Yang. 2009. "Community Health Service Centers in China, Not Always Trusted by the Populations They Serve?" *China Economic Review* 20: 620–24.

Yangpu (District) Archives (YPA): 47-13-62 and 47-13-70.

Yangpu District Tuberculosis Prevention and Treatment Clinic (YDTPTC) (杨浦区结核病防治所). 1992. *Chronicle of the Yangpu District Tuberculosis Prevention and Treatment Clinic* (上海市杨浦区结核病防治所所志). Shanghai: n.p.

Ye, Xifu, Deyu Huang, Alan R. Hinman, and Robert L. Parker. 1982. "Introduction to Shanghai County." *American Journal of Public Health*. 72 (Supplement): 13–18.

Yin Zuze (殷祖泽), ed. 2000. *Shanghai Jing'an District Health Gazetteer* (上海市静安区卫生志). Shanghai: Jing'an District Health Bureau (上海市静安区卫生局).

Yip, Ka-che. 1995. *Health and National Reconstruction in GMD China: The Development of Modern Health Services, 1928–1937*. Ann Arbor, MI: Association for Asian Studies.

Yip, Winnie Chi-Man, William C. Hsiao, Wen Chen, Shanlian Hu, Jin Ma, and Alan Maynard. 2012. "Early Appraisal of China's Huge and Complex Health Care Reforms." *Lancet* 379: 833–42.

Young, Mary. 1984. "A Study of Barefoot Doctor's Activities in China." PhD dissertation, Public Health, Johns Hopkins University.

Yu Hui (郁蕙), ed. 2011. *Xinbin Town Gazetteer* (新宾镇志). Shanghai: Shanghai Dictionary Publishers (上海辞书).

Yu Hui, and Liu Qiong (郁蕙、刘琼), eds. 2012. *Shihudang Town Gazetteer* (石湖荡镇志). Shanghai: Shanghai Dictionary Publishers (上海辞书).

Zhan, Shaohua. 2011. "What Determines Migrant Workers' Life Chances in Contemporary China? Hukou, Social Exclusion, and the Market." *Modern China* 37(3): 243–85.

Zhang, Daqing. 2014. "Changing Patterns of Disease and Longevity: The Evolution of Health in Twentieth Century Beijing." Pp. 32–50 in *Medical Transitions in Twentieth-Century China*, edited by B. Andrews and M. B. Bullock. Bloomington: University of Indiana Press.

Zhang Guogao (张国高). 1954. "How to Start TB Prevention Work among Workers?" (怎样开展工人防痨工作). *Mass Health* (大众卫生) 5: 170–74.

Zhang, Li. 2021. *The Origins of COVID-19: China and Global Capitalism*. Stanford, CA: Stanford University Press.

Zhang, Lixia, D. H. Tu, Y. S. An, and Donald A. Enarson. 2006. "The Impact of Migrants on the Epidemiology of Tuberculosis in Beijing, China." *International Journal of TB and Lung Disease* 10(9): 959–62.

Zhang, Yixia and Mark Elvin. 1998. "Environment and Tuberculosis in Modern China." Pp. 520–42 in *Sediments of Time*, edited by M. Elvin and T. Liu. Cambridge: Cambridge University Press.

Zhang Yurui (张玉瑞), ed. 1989. *Songjiang County Health Gazetteer* (松江县卫生志). Shanghai: Songjiang County Health Department Editorial Office (松江县卫生志编志办).

Zhao Hang (赵航), ed. 2011a. *Chedun Town Gazetteer* (车墩镇志). Shanghai: Shanghai Dictionary Publishers (上海辞书出版社).

Zhao Hang (赵航), ed. 2011b. *Xiaokunshan Town Gazetteer* (小昆山镇志). Shanghai: Shanghai Dictionary Publishers (上海辞书出版社).

Zhao, Yanlin, Shaofa Xu, Lixia Wang, Daniel P. Chin, Shengfen Wang, Guanglu Jiang, Hui Xia, Yang Zhou, Qiang Li, Xichao Ou, Yu Pang, Yuanyuan Song, Bing Zhao, Hongtao Zhang, Guangxue He, Jing Guo and Yu Wang. 2012. "National Survey of Drug-Resistant Tuberculosis in China." *New England Journal of Medicine* 366(23): 2161–70.

Zhi Zhong (志中). 1950. "Ministry of Health Decides to Promote BCG Vaccination in Major Cities" (卫生部决定在大城市推广卡介苗接种). *People's Daily* (人民日报), January 16.

Zhou, Xun. 2013. *Forgotten Voices of Mao's Great Famine, 1958–1962: An Oral History*. New Haven, CT: Yale University Press.

Zhou, Xun. 2020. *The People's Health: Health Intervention and Delivery in Mao's China, 1949–1983*. Montreal: McGill-Queen's University Press.

Zhu, Sui, Lan Xia, Shicheng Yu, Saobing Chen, and Juying Zhang. 2017. "The Burden and Challenges of Tuberculosis in China: Findings from the Global Burden of Disease Study." *Scientific Reports* 7: 14601.

Zhu, Yu. 2008. "The Resurgence of Shanghai and Its Demographic and Employment Changes in the 1990s." Pp. 251–83 in *Mega-Urban Regions in Pacific Asia: Urban Dynamics in a Global Era,* edited by G. Jones and M. Douglass. Singapore: National University of Singapore Press.

Index

Page numbers in bold refer to figures and tables.

Academia Sinica, 65
acquired immunodeficiency syndrome
    (AIDS), 8–9, 11–12, 179
active case finding (ACF). *See* case
    finding
Ai Jiong, 172–73
Anhui Province, 136, 151, 171
antibiotic resistance. *See* drug resistance
antibiotic treatment (for TB), 3, 6,
    10–11, **15**, 49, 71, 77–78, 83, 95–96,
    99, 102–3, 113, 120–25, 133, 137,
    151–52, 161, 163, 165–71. *See also*
    DOTS
anti-spitting, 41, 90–92; campaigns, 57,
    59; posters, **91–92**; spittoon, 90, 93
anti-tuberculosis movement, 26, 64, 71
anti-tuberculosis organizations, 28–30,
    40–41, 53, 64. *See also* NATAC, NTA,
    SATA

Bacillus Calmette Guerin. *See* BCG
Bamako Initiative, 13
Baoshan District, 16, 113, 138
barefoot doctors (BFDs), 6–7, 127–28,
    130–36, 139, 142, 147, 173–74;
    advantages, 132; limitations, 6,
    132–33; training, 6, 132
Barnes, David, 64
Barnes, Nicole Elizabeth, 5
Battle of Shanghai, 48
BCG vaccine, 8–10, 38, 49, 71, 84–85,
    90, 108, 113–16, 126, 136–38, 140;
    boosters, 113–15; in maternity wards,

114–15, 126; nurses, 114; rates, 85,
    113–15, 138; school vaccination, 115,
    126
beriberi, 35
biomedicine, 47, 51, 84, 100, 120
branch health offices (BHOs), 33–34, 37,
    62
Brazelton Mary Augusta, 116
Brehmer, Hermann, 30
brigade clinics, 6, 127–31, 134, 147, 157
Bu Liping, 51
Buhkman, Gene, 161

Canton Hospital, 64
case finding (for TB), 1, 6, 8, 17, 21, 78,
    83, 89, 96, 103, 107–8, 113, 124, 133,
    139–40, 162, 176, 181; active (ACF),
    15, 71–72, 77, 93–96, 118–20, 137,
    139; enhanced, 116, 175; passive,
    15, 119, 139, 162. *See also* X-ray and
    radiography
casual labor, 3, 7, 154–55. *See also*
    informal labor
Center for Disease Control (CDC), 18,
    144–45, 160, 168, 175
Central Epidemic Prevention Bureau,
    32–33
Changning District, 113, 175
Chendun town, 129, 143
Chengzhong Hospital, 62–63, 72, 107
chest x-ray. *See* X-ray
Chiang Kai-shek, 50
Child Labor Commission, 43–44

Index

China Anti-Tuberculosis Association (CATA). *See* National Anti-Tuberculosis Association of China

China Medical Association (CMA), 33–34, 94; Tuberculosis Conference, 53

China Medical Board (CMB), 33

China Medical Missionary Association (CMMA), 32–34

Chinese City, 27, 55

Chinese Communist Party (CCP), 4–5; 1949–89 policies, 5, 78–85, 99–103, 106, 129; policies after 1990, 7, 17

Chinese Health Bureau, 52, 55

Chinese medicine, 100, 172; for treating TB, 101–2, 163

cholera, 6, 35–37, 44, 50–51, 55, 71, 106; vaccination, 47, 71

Chongming County/island, 16, 135–36

Christmas seals, 29, 60

Chu, Henry, 46

Chuansha County, 113, 134–36, 138

collective owned enterprises (COEs), 79, 111, 124, 175; restructuring, 7, 153–55

collectivization, 85, 105; rural, 3, 6, 128–29

commune hospital, 129–30, 134, 139. *See also* town(ship) hospital

community health centers (CHCs), 20, 156–57, 160

compliance with medical advice, 9, 11–12, 121–22, 125, 139–40, 143, 160, 163; and drug resistance, 11–12, 151; enforcement in work units, 6, 81, 88–89, 103–4, 108, 117, 125, 140

cooperative medical system (CMS), 3, 6–7, 22, 130–34, 137, 139–44, 146–47, 158–59; new cooperative medical system (NSMS), 7, 144, 147, 159

Coordinating Committee for TB Control, 70–72, 77–78

cotton mills/factories, 18, 20, 58, 79, 112, 120–21

county hospitals, 129–30, 134, 139

COVID-19, 1, 3, 10, 14, 22, 56, 177, 179, 181

Cui Yitian, 96, 100

Cultural Revolution, 111, 115, 118–20, 131, 136–38

David Gregg Hospital for Women, 64

Davis, Mike, 179

Davis, Noel, 27, 37

Deng Xiaoping, 4, 17

Ding Fubao and Huikang, 63

dispensaries, 41–42

direct observed therapy (DOTS), 143, 160–63, 172–74, 176

drug-resistant tuberculosis, 11–12, 133, 151–52, 158, 161, 164, 170–72; extremely drug-resistant (XDR)-TB, 11, 172

dysentery, 35, 50

East China Normal University, 65, 100

educational campaign. *See* health education and TB prevention

extrapulmonary tuberculosis, 161, 164, 167, 169–70, 172

factory clinics and hospitals, 101, 111–12, 156, 168. *See also* infirmaries

factory doctors, 94, 112–13, 122–23, 145. *See also* workplace doctors

Fang, Xiaoping, 128, 13

Farmer, Paul, 12

Fengxian County/District, 19, 128, 131, 138–39, 143

Fifth National Cotton Factory, 77–78, 83, 88

First Five-Year Plan, 96, 99–100, 113

floating population, 154

Foucault, Michel, 34

Four Pest Elimination (除四害), 90, 93

French Concession, 27, 48–49, 55–56, 59, 62; French Municipal Council, 49, 69

fundamental causes theory, 9. *See also* social determinants of health

Fudan University, 107, 153

gastrointestinal illness, 35, 109–10. *See also* cholera and dysentery
gazetteers, 18, 103, 138–39, 142
germ theory of disease, 4
Gini coefficient, 17
global city, 3, 14–15, 17, 155
global health, 14, 113, 125, 177–79, 181; global health emergency, 8, 160
Gong You-Long, 143
government insurance system (GIS), 111, 157–58
Grant, John, 52
grassroots health facilities, 78, 107, 111–13. *See also* brigade clinic, factory clinic, school health clinics and hospitals, street-level health facilities and personnel, workplace clinic
Greater Shanghai Plan, 52
great famine, 130
Great Leap Forward, 6, 105, 107–9, 111, 113, 115, 117–21, 123, 125, 129
gross value of industrial output (GVIO), 16, 106, 130, 134, 142
Guomindang (GMD, 国民党), 4, 21, 46–50, 70–71, 73, 79, 81, 180; vision for health 4, 47, 50–52, 103, 178, 180

Hangzhou, 128
Harbin, 31, 172
health behavior, 9, 21, 93, 96, 103; health behavioral change, 50–51, 56, 59, 81, 90, 116; control of, 27, 41, 50, 81, 89–90, 103
health bureau, GMD Era (Chinese), 52, 55; post-1949, 83, 114, 131. *See also* Chinese Health Bureau, Shanghai Health Bureau
health-care system, three-tiered, 160; reform, 13, 143, 156–57, 163; rural, 129–30; urban, 111–13. *See also* CMS
health department. *See* SMC Health Department

health education, 6, 8–10, 21, 33–34, 50–51, 52, 78, 85–86, 115–16, 158, 162; TB-specific, 8, 29, 44, 51, 56–61, 70–71, 73, 86–89, 95, 100–101, 113, 116–18, 122, 136, 158, 160, 173
Health News (健康报), 78, 101
Health Officer's Report (HOR), 34–36, 38, 41
health promotion, 5, 78–79, 109, 146, 169
health stations, in Northern China, 34, 52; rural Shanghai, 130, 140, 147; Shanghai urban subdistrict, 37, 52, 111, 123
Henriot, Christian, 81
Ho, Denise, 87
Hongqiao Commune, 134–35, 143
Hongqiao (Hungjao 虹桥) Sanitarium/ Sanatorium, 62–63, 71
Hospital Building and Equipment Fund Campaign, 67
household registration (*hukou*), 10, 15–16, 80, 123
Howlett, Johnathon, 80–81
Huang, Philip, 129, 141
Huangpu River, 14, 17
Huashan Hospital, 72 (footnote), 102
Hudong Workers' Cultural Palace, 117
Hu Hongji (胡鸿基), 52
hukou. *See* residence permit
Huizenga, Lee S., 46, 48, 55, 65, 67
human development index, 17
human immunodeficiency virus (HIV), 8, 11–12. *See also* AIDS
Hung, Chang-tai, 86
Huyangqiao village, 129, 142
Hyde, Sandra, 174
hygiene campaigns, 49, 84–85, 90, 101, 109. *See also* health education programs
hygienic modernity, 52
hypercolonial, 27, 34

immunization, 33, 83, 107, 115–16, 132, 135–37; cholera, 37; smallpox, 37, 71. *See also* vaccination and BCG

Index

incidence (other diseases), 11, 35–36, 109; TB, 11, 13, 18, 39, 42, 54–55, 99, 110–11, 118

indiscriminate spitting, 41, 57, 90, 110, 116

industrialization, and disease control, 26, 28, 98, 106, 110, 125; de-industrialization, 153; in rural areas, 141

industrial production, 105–6; link with infectious disease, 105; rural 141. *See also* GVIO

infirmaries (workplace-built), 77–78, 84, 99–100, 120–21, 139. *See also* Fifth National Cotton Factory

influenza, 35–36

informal labor, 58, 154, 159, 179. *See also* casual labor

inoculation. *See* vaccination and BCG

international health, cooperation, 31–33, 44, 49–50, 70, 177–78; fellowship, 52; protocols, 85, 108, 113, 180

International Settlement, 26–27, 35–36, 40, 42, 48, 55, 56, 59, 62, 68; health department, 27; ratepayers, 25–26, 29, 38, 40. *See also* SMC

International Tuberculosis Awareness Day, 145, 175

iron rice bowl (铁饭碗), 5, 80, 155

isolation of disease sufferers (e.g., COVID and Manchurian Plague), 1, 4, 32, 145; of TB sufferers, 3, 10, **15**, 25–26, 29, 38–41, 44–45, 48, 53–54, 56, 61–70, 78, 96, 99–103, 113–14, 120–21, 137, 181. *See also* infirmaries, sanatoria

isoniazid, 10–11, 101–3; isoniazid preventive therapy (IPT), 8–10

Japanese Occupation, 21, 47–48, 54, 61–73, 82–83, 103, 106, 146, 181

Jiading Country/District, 16, 113, 128, 136, 138, 168; Tuberculosis Prevention and Treatment Clinic, 140–41

Jiangsu Province, 82, 95, 141, 171

Jiaotong University, 60, 100, 107, 121, 142

Jing'an District, 19, 62, 100

Jinshan County, 128, 136–39

Johns Hopkins Homewood Institutional Review Board, 20

Johnston, William, 64

Jordan, J. H., 27, 48

June 26th Directive, 130, 135–37

Kang Youwei, 51

King's Daughters Society, 49

Khrushchev, Nikita Sergeyevich, 105, 109

Koch, Erin, 11, 13

Koch, Robert, 3, 28, 30

Kurhaus, 30

labor insurance system (LIS), 111, 157–58

laid-off workers, 20, 159, 168, 176

Lam, Tong, 34

land reform, 128–29

League of Nations Health Organization (LHNO), 32–33, 50, 178

Lei, Sean Hsiang-Lin, 53

Li Peng, 17

Li Ting'an (李廷安), 52

life expectancy, 11, 13, 17–18, 125, 179

Linsheng (霖生) Hospital, 66

literacy rates, 58, 88

Liu Ying, 166–67

"lonely island" (孤岛) period, 48

lost labor due to illness, 77, 96, 109–10, 116, 125

Lu Jinling, 90, 93

Lu Xun, 51

Madras Study, 96, 120

malnutrition. *See* social determinants of health

Manchurian Plague, 4, 26, 31–34, 44

Mao Zedong, 78, 105, 109, 130, 135–37

market socialism, 122, 177–78

masking, 1, 3, 31, 36, 56

mass mobilization, **15**, 47, 51, 84, 89, 105

mass radiography, 49, 93–95, 113, 118–19, 137. *See also* case finding and x-ray

McKeown, Thomas, 10, 54
measles, 35
medical protests (医闹), 159, 180
midwives, 5, 51, 132
migrant, 1, 7, 16, 58, 154–55, 162, 172–74, 176; population, 3, 154, 162; workers, 159, 167, 176
migration, 14, 16, 22, 80, 82, 128, 153–55, 162; control, **15**; structural barriers to, 7, 10, 81; TB risk, 11–12
Minhang District, 128, 134. *See also* Shanghai County
Ministry of Health, 50, 84–85,102, 114, 137
mobile medical teams, 135–37
mobile x-ray vehicles/units. *See* active case finding, radiography and x-ray
modernity, 25–26, 52, 179
modernization, 4, 26, 28, 31–32, 45, 47, 177; socialist modernization, 5, 109, 177–78
monitoring, health-related, 6, 20, 78, 89, 93–96, 103, 118, 158, 161; environmental sanitation, 52; peer-on-peer, 89–90, 96, 103; statistical, 34, 36 50, 94, 96, 103
mortality, 13, 34–37, **55**; TB-related, 13, 18, 22, 25, 34, 38, 42, 53–56, 70, 82–83, 96, 99, 104, 125, 133, 139–40
multi-drug resistant tuberculosis (MDR-TB). *See* drug-resistant TB
Municipal Anti-TB Work Representative Meeting, 88, 93–94
Municipal Council Sanitorium, 25–27, 38–42, 62–63, 67–68
Municipal Health Department. *See* SMC Health Department
Municipal Isolation Hospital, 25, 39–40, 44–45, 61

Nakajima, Cheiko, 47, 49
Nanhui County, 136, 138
Nanjing, 46–48, 62, 95, 100, 171; Nanjing Decade, 4, 46–47, 49–50, 57, 61; Nanjing Government, 44, 47, 61

Nankai University, 85
Nanpu Bridge, 17
National Anti-Tuberculosis Association of China (NATAC), 30, 53, 57–58, 60–62, 71, 137
National Health Administration, 50–51
national health reconstruction program, 4, 47, 50–53, 56, 60, 85, 180
National Tuberculosis Association (NTA), 28–30
neighborhood committees, 109, 118, 122–23, 126, 181. *See also* residents' committees
neighborhood hospitals, 122
neoliberal policies, 12–15, 179; approach to health, 13
New Life Movement, 50, 53, 180
nurse/nursing, 5, 40–41, 121–23, 135–36, 140, 145, 157, 160; BCG nurses, 114; public health nurses, 22, 123, 125; standardization of training, 51; TB prevention nurses, 89, 100–101

Ocean Shipping Supervision Bureau, 99
Opium War, 14
outpatient treatment. *See* treatment of TB

Patriotic Hygiene Campaign (爱国卫生运动), 84–85, 90
Peking Union Medical College (PUMC), 33, 52
People's Daily (人民日报), 85
People's Republic of China (PCR), 4, 16
permanent employment, 7; elimination of, 7, 22, 153–55, 175
personal protective equipment, 1
Perry, Elizabeth, 89
plague, 35–36, 44, 50–51; bubonic, 36. *See also* Manchurian Plague
planned economy, 80, 153
Pleasant Goat (喜羊羊), 175
pneumonic plague, 31–32. *See also* Manchurian plague
pneumothorax, 64–65, 70

population of Shanghai, 14–16, 81–82; migrant, 3, 154; rural communes, 129, 134, 143; stabilization, 5, 16, 78; strengthening, 31, 99; vulnerable, 25, 42–43

prevalence of infectious disease, 11; of TB 11, 34, 40, 42, 50, 71, 93–96, 99, 104–6, 115, 124–25; in rural counties, 127–28, 133, 138–40; in Xuhui and Yangpu Districts, 124

preventative health (care)/medicine, 13, 50, 71, 127, 145, 160; in rural areas 22, 127, 130, 132

prevention programs (for TB), 21, 29, 41, 56–61, 70–71, 78, 83–89, 103, 113–18, 125, 175. *See also* BCG

primary health care, 6, 12, 81, 132, 156–57, 179

primary prevention (of TB), 116, 118, 125

Private Shanghai Hospital, 80, 123

privatization, 7, 12–13, 22, 153–55, 175

production brigades, 3, 6 7, 127, 129, 131–34, 136, 141, 146–47, 155, 159

Progressive Era/movement, 26, 29, 44

public health, 1, 3–4, 6, 9, 18, 20, 22, 26, 29, 31–35, 51–53, 59, 73, 81, 83–84, 86, 88–90, 93, 96, 100, 103, 106, 125, 145, 155–56, 178; infrastructure, 4, 14, 22, 81; interventions, 10, 27–28, 33, 54, 181; nurses, 22, 123, 125; system, 6–7, 10, 12, 14 22, 155, 180; work, 21, 31, 33, 73, 178

public health posters. *See* Shanghai Anti-Tuberculosis Association posters

Public Health Service (French), 49

Public Shanghai Hospital, 80

Pudong District, 16–17, 134. *See also* Chuansha County

Putuo District, 113, 175

Qingpu County/District, 138

radiography. *See* mass radiography

Red Cross, 65, 72

refugee, 54, 60–61, 73; camp, 60, 65; Second Red Cross Refugee Treatment Hospital, 65-**66**

residence permit (户口), 7, 10, 15–16, 123, 154, 180. *See also* household registration

residents' committee, 20, 22, 89, 100, 118. *See also* neighborhood committee

Revised Law of the Prevention and Control on Infectious Diseases, 156, 177

Riis, Jacob, 29

Rockefeller Foundation, 32–33, 50, 178; Rockefeller Foundation International Health Board Fellowship, 52

Rogaski, Ruth, 27

Rothman, Shelia, 30

Russian Orthodox Confraternity's Hospital, 64

sanatoria/sanatorium, 3, 10, **15**, 29–31, 38–42, 56, 62–63, 67, 68, 71, 72, 99 101, 120, 138, 171; movement, 26, 29–30, 38

Saranac Lake Sanitorium, 28–29

scarlet fever, 35, 50, 55

schistosomiasis, 6, 84, 166

school health, BCG administration, 85, 113–16, 126; campaigns 50–51, 57, 59–60, 70–71, 86, 90–**91**, 93–96; 109, 117, 160; clinics and hospitals, 20, 145, 156, 166, 175; conference on, 34

scientific medicine, 51, 61. *See also* Western medicine

Second Sino-Japanese War, 47

serve the people, 6, 137

severe acute respiratory syndrome (SARS), 1–2, 8, 14, 156, 177, 179, 180

sexually transmitted infections, 6, 11

Shandong Province, 102–3

Shanghai Anti-Tuberculosis Association (SATA, 上海防痨协会), 1–**2**, 46, 48–49, 53, 55–56, 58–61, 63–73, 79, 86–88, 91–93, 95–98, 178; American Committee of, 71; annual reports,

54, 60, 65–67, 86; essay contest, 60, 146; hospital superintendent, 46, 62; Medical Committee, 63, 69; posters, 1–2, 86–88, 90, **91–92**, 95–96, **97–98**; First Hospital, 99; Shanghai Hospital, 46, 48, 65–**66**, 80, 107; Tuberculosis Hospital, 65, 67–70; preventive educational campaigns, 58–60, 86–88, 90

Shanghai Coordinating Committee for Tuberculosis Control, 70–73, 77

Shanghai County, 113, 133–36, 138–39, 141, 143. *See also* Minhang District

Shanghai First Iron and Steel Plant, 122, 167

Shanghai Health Bureau, 83, 114, 131

Shanghai Library, 107

Shanghai Medical College, 70, 93, 100, 107, 136, 143

Shanghai Municipal Anti-TB Work Representative Meeting, 88, 93–94

Shanghai Municipal Archives (SMA), 38

Shanghai Municipal Council (SMC), 27, 32–44, 48, 50, 52, 56, 59, 61–63, 69, 178; Annual Meeting of the Ratepayers, 25; health commissioner, 39, 48; Health Department, 32, 34, 36–37, 39, 50, 52, 56, 178; ratepayers, 38, 40; Sanatorium, 25–27, 38–42, 62–63, 67–68. *See also* International Settlement

Shanghai Municipal TB Prevention Committee, 88

Shanghai Pulmonary Hospital, 107, 121. *See also* Chengzhong Hospital

Shanghai Smelting Plant, 109–10

Shanghai University, 166, 170

Sheshan town, 129, 142

Sidel, Ruth, and Victor, 6, 127, 132, 143

Sinclair, Upton, 29

smallpox, 35, 37, 45, 50, 55, 71; immunization, 71; vaccines, 35, 37

social control, 7, 32, 41–42, 50, 80–83, 178, 181; control of health behaviors,

27, 41, 50, 56, 81, 89–90, 103; of prisoners, 42–43; of respiratory disease sufferers, 4, 26, 32; state control, 34, 85–86, 96, 106, 178, 181; in work-units, 7, 80–83, 89, 104, 181

social determinants of health, 1, 5, 9–10, 21, 25–26, 29, 32, 39–40, 42–44, 58, 64–65, 73, 82, 109, 162, 177–79; housing, 1, 5, 10, 25, 29, 39, 42, 84, 155, 173; (mal)nutrition, 1, 5, 8–10, 25, 29, 43, 54, 64, 68, 84, 99, 139, 177; poverty, 1, 9–10, 12, 40, 52, 58; quality of life, 26, 84, 155, 179; standard of living, 10, 54, 84, 103

social distancing, 8, 10, 31, 56

socialization, 85–86; health socialization, 81, 82, 83, 86, 93, 116; resocialization, 85; reverse socialization, 93

Songjiang County/District, 128–31, 138–42; Tuberculosis Prevention and Treatment Clinic 113, 138, 140

Soon, Wayne, 84

Southern Tour, 4, 17

Soviet (health) model, 70, 82; post-Soviet collapse, 11, 13, 161

Soviet Union, 70, 105, 161

spittoons, 90, 93. *See also* anti-spitting

sputum smear test, 120, 122, 161

St. Luke's Hospital, 65

Stanley, Arthur, 27, 39–41

State Council, 17

state-owned enterprise (SOE), 13, 111, 124, 151, 162, 166–69, 175; GMD state enterprises, 79; restructuring, 7, 153–55, 160

stigma, 1, 11, 180; TB stigma, 170–71

street-level health facilities and personnel, 115, 118–19, 122–23, 125

streptomycin, 10–11, 69, 102

Strong Ox, 144

Suzhou Creek, 20, 48

symptoms of TB, 29, 57–58, 139; education about, 8, 70, 84, 86, 113, 116, 139, 175

Index 215

Taiyuan Municipal Tuberculosis Prevention and Treatment Hospital, 95

Takagi, K., 69

temporary work. *See* casual labor and informal labor

textile factories/mills, 58, 81, 106–7, 121, 166–67, 169; working conditions, 43–44, 168–69, 186. *See also* Fifth National Cotton Factory

Tianjin, 16

Tillman, Margaret, 49, 60, 65

Tongji University, 100, 107

total institution, 6, 43, 81

town(ship) hospital, 142

township and village enterprise (TVEs), 7, 22, 141–44

trachoma, 51, 109

traditional Chinese medicine. *See* Chinese medicine

treatment of tuberculosis, nutritional, 39, 43, 77, 84, 99, 102; outpatient, 41, 44, 49, 51, 61 62, 65, 67 68, 72, 93, 96, 100, 112. *See also* antibiotic treatment, Chinese medicine, infirmaries, isolation of disease sufferers, and sanatoria

treaty ports, 36, 69

Trudeau, Edward Livingston, 29

tuberculin skin tests, 115, 138

tuberculosis (TB) control network, 6, 20, 22, 80, 109, 112, 122, 126–27, 160

tuberculosis prevention and treatment hospitals and clinics, 95, 102; county, 113, 138, 140–41; municipal, 93, 108, 112, 114, 124, 138; district, 20, 22, 106–7, 112–14, 116–19, 125, 135, 138, 140, 160, 175. *See also* Jiading County, Songjiang County, Xuhui District, Yangpu District

tuberculosis question, 25, 40

typhoid, 35, 50, 55, 71

typhus, 29

United Nations Development Program (UNDP), 17

university district, 145–46

university entrance exam (高考), 145

vaccination/vaccine, 3, 8–9, 35, 37–38, 47, 49, 52, 56, 71, 78, 85, 103, 113–15, 136, 179; cholera, 47, 71; COVID-19, 3, 56; smallpox, 35, 37, 71. *See also* BCG

venereal disease, 33. *See also* sexually transmitted infections (STIs)

village doctors, 140, 142–43, 147, 179

Wang Hongtie, 90–91, 101–2

Warlord period, 26

War of Resistance against the Japanese, 4, 47, 49

welfare, 4–5, 7, 22, 29, 49–50, 108, 141, 154, 179–80

Wenzhou, 106, 165, 170, 181, 185

Western medicine, 6, 26, 33, 51, 63, 99, 102 3, 133, 136, 139

Wing On textiles, 59

workplace clinics and hospitals, 6–8, 81, 86, 111–13, 118, 120, 123, 145, 156, 160, 163, 166, 168. *See also* brigade clinics, factory clinics

workplace doctors, 6, 8, 22, 112–13, 120–23, 125, 140, 145, 163, 173; school health personnel, 94, 113, 115, 122. *See also* barefoot doctors, factory doctors

work-unit (单位) system (WUS), 3; benefits, 3, 5–6, 10, 80–81, 83–85, 107–8, 111–12, 173, 179; creation, 78–80, 108; dismantling, 7, 151–55, 174; role in disease control, 3, 6–9, 12–14, 20–22, 77–78, 81, 86, 93–104, 113–22, 124–26, 160, 162, 176, 180–82; rural equivalent, 6, 140, 144–47; surveillance function, 78, 80–81, 121, 181; systemic inequalities, 112, 119, 123–26, 180

World Bank, 13, 125, 161
World Health Organization (WHO), 6–7, 70, 85, 108, 160
World Trade Organization (WTO), 17
World War I, 26, 38
World War II, 73, 178. *See also* Japanese Occupation
Wu Liande (Wu Lien-teh, 伍连德), 31
Wu Shaoqing (吴绍青), 70, 72, 89, 94, 99
Wu Tiecheng (Wu Te-chen 吴铁城), 53

Xiaokunshan Town, 130, 142
Xinbin Town, 142
Xinhua Bookstore, 100
Xinhua Central Hospital, 121
Xinhua News Agency, 131
Xinqiao Town, 130, 142
X-ray (chest), 46, 64, 65, 68, 71–72, 77, 118; slides, 113, 118, 120; vehicle/ mobile unit, 93–96, **97**, 101, 103, 119, 126, 160, 162. *See also* mass radiography and case finding
Xuhui District, 107, 124, 133, 135; Central Hospital, 63; TB prevalence, 124; Tuberculosis Prevention and Treatment Clinic, **66**, 80, 107–8, 113–15, 118–25, 135–36

Yang Xuegong, 169
Yangpu District, 48, 62, 107–8, 110–12, 117, 120–22, 124–25, 153, 156; Central Hospital, 121, 169; industrial restructuring, 153–54; TB incidence, 110; TB prevalence, 124, Tuberculosis Prevention and Treatment Clinic, 110–11, 113, 115–17, 120–22, 124, 136
Yangtze River, 14, 35
Yip, Ka-che, 88
Young Men's Christian Association (YMCA), 32–34, 60
Yu Ya Ching TB Sanitarium, 62
YWCA Nurses Association, 34

Zhabei District, 36, 47–48, 54, 113, 124
Zhejiang Province, 82, 128, 136
Zhongshan Hospital, 70, 102, 107–8, 114, 120, 136, 138
Zhou, Xun, 133